INTRODUCTION

While it may seem like a strange idea, 'to lose fat, eat more fat', people are beginning to awaken to the idea that it is carbs (mostly processed carbs and sugar) that are the actual cause of rising health problems around the world (such as type 2 diabetes).

In recent years, studies have shown that the benefits of a Ketogenic Diet include:

- Accelerated fat loss
- Lower cholesterol
- Lower blood sugar
- Increased energy levels and vitality
- Improved mental focus (ketogenic diets were initially used for epilepsy)

If you follow a Ketogenic Diet then you will experience the health benefits. However, for some (if not most), the initial excitement fades as you eat the same burger with no bun for the third time this week; become tired of constantly looking at food labels; feel awkward in social situations just wanting to eat something 'normal' for a change or the whole diet just becomes tiresome as you have to eat exactly 1981 calories every day, of which 394 must come from Wagyu Beef.

I want to provide you with not just another diet which you must follow religiously, otherwise it will not work, but a diet where the principles are a sound method of adapting the diet to your lifestyle and not the other way around. Yes, it will still require work, dedication, and label reading (in the beginning at least), but once you have the knowledge and experience, you'll progress from beginner to master and you can begin to adapt the Ketogenic Diet to how you live your life. This is what the guide promises to give you.

The 100 recipes will keep you from bland food and boredom. None of the recipes are 'gourmet' and they don't require ingredients from a remote village in South America or liquid nitrogen for preparation. The recipes are intended to be 'everyday'; easy to find ingredients; easy to prepare (less than 25 minutes) but still tasty. All the recipes include detailed nutritional information (to save you from looking at all the labels).

I also realize starting a diet can be hard. Procrastination is often a killer to many health goals. As a bonus, I created the Quick Start Guide and 7 Day Meal Planner. This is so you can read the short guide and start your diet *today!* More on this in the next chapter.

Once again, thank you for buying this book, and I hope you will give me the privilege of helping you create your own sustainable lifestyle on the Ketogenic Diet.

YOUR ROAD MAP TO SUCCESS

This book is intended to be the most comprehensive guide you can find, however, an overload of information can be daunting. To make navigation easier, below is your road map to the book and a healthier you.

Part I - Ketogenic Overview

This covers the basics of the diet, the benefits, and what to expect.

Part 2 – Step by Step Guide to Achieving Ketosis and Fat Loss

As they say, the devil is in the details, and this is where we go into detail on the steps required to achieve ketosis and fat loss.

Part 3 – Adapting the Diet to Your Life – (No More Calorie Counting)

You will learn the 80% Approach to dieting and how to adapt the diet to your life. And, of course, how to stop calorie counting altogether.

Part 4 - Preparing to Succeed

This section prepares you for the be start possible. We'll cover key preparations, how to stay on track, and tips to achieve your health goals. Also included is a 7-day meal plan to make your first week as easy as possible.

Part 5 - 100 Delicious Recipes (Need I say more?)

BONUS FALL & WINTER SERIES

Thank you for downloading the book, I really appreciate it. I would like to return the favor. I am giving away the 'Fall & Winter Mini Series'. These are my favorite fall & winter recipes including quick and easy meals, brunches, desserts, ice cream and more.

Simply visit the link below to get your free copy:

http://geni.us/Keto100Land

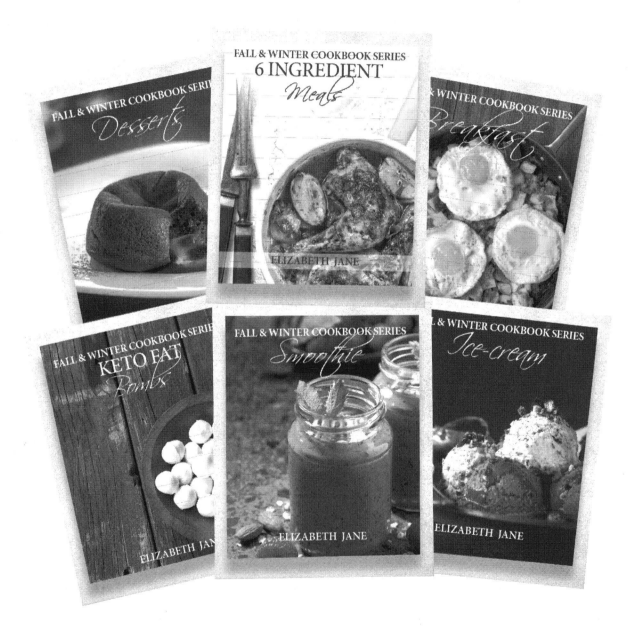

TABLE OF CONTENTS

PART I KETOGENIC DIET OVERVIEW

WHAT IS A KETOGENIC DIET?

Our body's metabolism has evolved much less quickly than modern technology. In the past, we had to hunt for our meals and we would often go without food for days or weeks at a time. As a result, our bodies stored as much of its energy reserves as possible for when it was needed. The body became extremely efficient at taking any excess energy (from food) and storing it for later (as fat). When food became scarce, the body would switch from using food as its main source of energy to the fat reserves.

However, in modern life, food is far more plentiful but excess energy is still be stored as fat. Modern life has exacerbated this by producing foods rich in carbohydrates (which are utilized more quickly by the body), and lowering the need for physical activity, hence excess energy (more calories are consumed than expended) is more abundant and consequently more energy is stored (usually as fat).

The concept of the ketogenic diet is that it takes advantage of your body's natural system that uses fat for fuel. By switching to a low carbohydrate diet, your body adapts – unable to utilize the readily available source of carbohydrate that was once available to it. Instead, it begins to use both existing and new stores of fat as its energy source. This is known as a state of **ketosis**.

When we are on a diet containing sufficient amounts of carbohydrate, they are broken down into glucose which is used for energy. However, when carbs are restricted, our liver starts to produce ketones (also known as ketone bodies). These are transported from the liver to other tissues where they can be reconverted by enzymes in the body to produce energy.

Your aim is to reach a state of Ketosis. This is the stage where you are fueled by fat. There is a large difference between normal ketone levels and being in ketosis. Thus it will be a big change for your body.

BENEFITS OF A KETOGENIC DIET

Lower blood sugar and insulin levels – helping to prevent and manage diabetes

When carbs are consumed, they are broken down into glucose, increasing the blood sugar levels. The body responds by releasing insulin (to lower blood sugar levels). Unfortunately, if you overload your body continuously with sugar (as a result insulin), the cells in your body becomes resistant to the insulin. Your body's natural process to reduce your blood sugar is reduced. Hence, your blood sugar remains unnaturally high. This is type II diabetes.

So what's the simple solution to bringing your blood sugar down? Do not eat carbs (which produce the sugar). One study suggested diabetics on a low carb diet can reduce their insulin dosage by 50% (1).

Lower blood sugar also results in feeling better. Remember when you have a big lunch then feel sleepy for the rest of the afternoon? That was because of a spike in your blood sugar.

Suppressing your appetite

On a ketogenic diet, you feel fuller, which means you crave food (including junk food), far less. This then becomes a simple equation, if you feel like eating less, you eat less. Eating less ultimately leads to weight loss.

Greater fat loss – particularly the stubborn belly fat

Potentially one of the best benefits of the ketogenic diet is increased fat loss around the stomach area. Shedding this visceral fat around the mid region was always something I struggled with and I began to see a significant reduction in fat on a ketogenic diet. One study which compared a low fat and a low carb diet was surprised at this finding:

Both between and within group comparisons revealed a distinct advantage of a VLCK (low carb) over a LF (low fat) diet for weight loss, total fat loss, and trunk fat loss for men' (2)

They also highlighted the trunk loss in women, but it was not as significant as within men (women tend to store fat more proportionally around the body).

The loss of visceral (internal) fat helps to reduce the chances of diabetes and general health problems in the future.

Lower levels of triglycerides

Triglycerides are fat in your blood. You may think this is a bad thing, but they are needed to provide energy around the body. If you have too many of them, however, your body saves them for a rainy day somewhere around your body as fat. High levels also lead to a higher chance of diabetes and heart disease.

One of the biggest contributing factors to high levels is simple sugars. Cutting out these sugars reduces your triglyceride levels.

Increase in good cholesterol and a decrease in bad cholesterol

At one point, all cholesterol was considered bad, however within recent years it has been proven that there is good and bad cholesterol.

LDL (low density lipoprotein) is the bad stuff, while HDL (high density lipoprotein) is the good stuff.

HDL carries cholesterol from the rest of the body for processing, where it is used or 'thrown away'. LDL can clot and form fatty deposits, blocking arteries (contributing to heart conditions and increased blood pressure).

Studies have shown one of the best ways to increase HDL levels and reduce LDL levels is a high fat diet.

Increased mental focus

Low carb diets were one of the earliest forms of treatment for epilepsy (until more effective drugs were developed). The diet is also now being explored as a way to treat and stave off Alzheimer's and Parkinson's disease.

Fatty acids (particularly omega 3 and 6) are considered beneficial for cognitive functioning and help you keep more focused and alert.

WHAT TO EXPECT ON A KETOGENIC DIET

The long term health benefits of a ketogenic diet have been well documented; lower blood pressure, lower cholesterol, lower triglycerides levels, fat loss, increased energy, greater mental acuity, better moods and improvements to the digestive system.

Over the first week or so, you should notice a sudden drop in weight as your body begins to adapt. In particular, your body will begin to retain less water (which is needed for a diet containing higher levels of carbohydrates). As such, you may feel thirsty and require a higher frequency of trips to the toilet!

During your first week, your body will undergo a sort of 'carb detox' which may result in you feeling subpar – this is sometimes referred to as the 'keto flu'. It should only last for a few days and is evidence that your body is shifting and changing for the better.

Tip – *If you do experience 'keto flu', perceive it as a positive and evidence that it is working - focus on the end outcome (fat loss etc.). It will only last a few days.*

Take care not to overdo it!

As with everything in life, too much of a good thing is often more harmful than good and things should never be taken to the extreme.

This is a very low carb diet, but not a **no carb** diet, as it will often be extremely difficult (if not impossible) to avoid all carbs completely.

Anything which is done in excess is a bad thing!

While it is extremely unlikely, there is a risk of ketoacidosis, when there are too many ketones released into the body and the blood becomes acidic. This is extremely unlikely to occur on this diet, as it is more commonly associated with poorly controlled type 1 diabetes or alcoholism. However, it is important to be aware of the symptoms which include; extreme tiredness, blurry vision, vomiting, dehydration and collapsing. If you experience any of these then consult your physician and increase your daily carbohydrates.

This can be easily avoided by ensuring that you do not go to extremes, (e.g. cutting all carbs completely) and follow the guidelines set out in this book.

The ketogenic diet should be part of a balanced lifestyle (diet and exercise). While eating 4kg of ice cream everyday adheres to the principles of a ketogenic diet (low carb / high fat), it is obviously not the best approach for a healthy lifestyle. It is important to ensure that your food choices are sufficient enough to provide you with a balanced diet. A specific breakdown of food types and amounts is provided later.

PART II – STEP BY STEP GUIDE TO ACHIEVING KETOSIS

PROCESS OVERVIEW

The below diagram is a simplified guide to this section.

1. **Calculate total calories needed** – This is vital. It's simple equation, if you are consuming more energy (calories) than you expend, then you will put on weight.
2. **Calculate macros** – This is the nuts and bolts, how many grams of carbs, fats and proteins do you need?
3. **Monitor / optimize** – One size does not fit all. You'll learn how to tailor the diet to your body and needs.

Steps to Ketosis

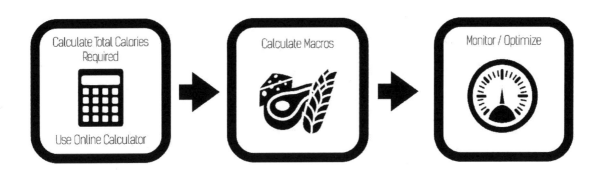

"Eat fresh and natural, if it lasts forever...It is probably not natural or fresh."

Anonymous

GETTING TO KNOW YOUR FOOD – WHAT TO EAT & WHAT TO AVOID

Before launching into the details of the ketogenic diet, it is important to understand some basic principles about eating well, which foods to eat, and which to avoid.

The general principle of the ketogenic diet is low carb, high fat, and adequate protein from good healthy sources. As mentioned before, calories come in lots of different forms, so a good start is to get to know what these are.

FATS

Pure fats come in their natural state from their original food. This includes animal fat, avocados, eggs, coconuts, seeds, nuts, olives, and fish fat.

Tampered fats are modified versions of the above like olive oil, butter, coconut butter, vegetable oils, and fish oils.

"Ugly" fats are further processed fats, such as trans-fats (which you've no doubt heard of!). Trans-fat foods are easy to identify these days because the word "hydrogenated" is included somewhere in the ingredients. That's partially, fully, or whatever kind of hydrogenated.

Ideally, most of your fats on a ketogenic diet should come from the family of pure fats, with some from the tampered fats. Try to avoid ugly fats entirely. There are too many different types of foods for me to provide a comprehensive list, but the easiest way to ensure you are mainly eating from the pure fats category is to ask yourself if it has been altered in anyway and to try to prepare the majority of your food from raw ingredients.

PROTEIN

Lean protein such as chicken, tuna, turkey - anything which is nearly all protein and nothing else.

Fatty protein such as eggs, most red meat, fatty fish, cottage cheese, etc.

Dairy which tends to be a combination of fat, carbs and protein.

There is no general rule regarding the above, and is provided more for knowledge and awareness. It is helpful knowing whether your food is a combination (fat / protein) or pure protein because it'll help you to balance your diet.

Tip - Dairy agrees with some people more than others. Once I removed dairy from my diet I felt far less bloated after meals and had more energy. Try with / without for one week and see how you feel.

CARBOHYDRATES

Ketogenic is a very low carbohydrate diet, but the aim is not to eliminate them completely.

Complex carbs come in two varieties gluten containing (wheat, rye, paste, bread etc.) and non-gluten containing (rice, potatoes, quinoa, beans etc.).

Simple carbs such as fruit

Vegetables – where possible try to eat fresh rather than frozen (I recommend these as they are high in vitamins, fiber and minerals).

"Ugly" carbs which are mostly processed sugars (think biscuits, sweets/candy etc.)

Try to stick to complex carbs with some simple carbs and at least one cup of vegetables every day. It goes without saying, avoid processed or ugly carbs as much as possible.

Tip - Consider toying with the gluten vs gluten free. I found my body reacted much better to gluten free foods (love quinoa!).

TOTAL CARBS VS NET CARBS

There is a debate about which to measure when on the diet for your calorie intake.

Total carbs is the total amount of all of the carbs that you eat. Net carbs, however, is total carbs minus fiber carbs.

This can be confusing, isn't a carb a carb? Not when it is not digested and goes straight through you.

The theory is that fiber is not digested, hence does not contain any calories and should not contribute towards your calorie count. However this has the added complexity of soluble vs insoluble fiber. Insoluble fiber (by definition) is not absorbed and has no calories, whereas soluble fiber (by definition) is absorbed.

Unfortunately, the science behind this is conflicting with several experts providing different views.

From my experience, net carbs worked best for me. And it is this which I recommend. The one caveat with this, is most food labels do not show net carbs, hence you will have to deduct the fiber from total carbs each time (and just assume most of the fiber is insoluble to make your life easier).

STEP 1 – CALCULATING TOTAL CALORIES REQUIRED

I did promise to show you a life without counting calories, however you need to learn the basics and put in some effort to begin with. You would not expect to be able to play guitar like Lenny Kravitz the first time you picked up a guitar. You need to learn the basics. And with experience comes the freedom of 'no more calorie counting'. So let's begin with the basics.

The general principle of the ketogenic diet is simple, eat very few carbs, high fat and adequate protein.

The approach that works best for you may differ from other members of your family or friends. For example, you may find weight loss occurs more efficiently with certain types of food and not others.

Below I present the recommended guidelines, with the caveat that there may be a little bit of trial and error to tweak the different numbers and food types in the first few weeks to see what is working and what is not. Try, if possible, to keep a diary so you can record any changes. I would recommend MyFitnessPal as a useful app for keeping track of what you are eating and changes to your weight and body composition.

Let's get into the specifics, what are the 'rules' of a ketogenic diet?

First, we need to know where we currently stand.

HOW MANY CALORIES DO I NEED A DAY?

Total calories needed to exist (calculating BMR)

The starting point for any diet is to know the number of calories you need per day just to exist, this is our basic metabolic rate (BMR). The calculation considers your age, gender, height, weight and activity level.

Visit the below link to easily work out your BMR.

http://geni.us/CalcBMR

This provides you with our theoretical 'maintenance' calorie intake. If you ate this number of calories a day you would neither gain nor lose weight.

I recommend using these numbers in the first 3-4 weeks as your 'benchmark'. Over the next few pages you'll learn how to adjust this number, by how much, and how often. But first we need to breakdown our calories further.

STEP 2 – CALCULATING MACROS

Macronutrient Breakdown

Most resources use percentages of total calories to provide guidance on the amount of carbs, proteins and fats (usually around 70% from fat, 20 % from protein and 10% from carbs). However, I do not believe the percentages are a useful starting point. Most recipes and packaged foods display proteins (for example) in grams and also makes assumptions that as we change weight we need more/fewer carbs (which may not be the case). I propose to work with grams instead.

- Carbs - 20 - 50 grams per day

    o Try 30 grams to begin with, see how you feel, and how you're progressing (see measuring results below).

- Protein - or 1.5 – 2.6 grams per pound (0.7 – 1.2 grams per kg) of body weight.

    o If your level of physical activity is high, go for the higher end as it will help to retain/ build muscle.

- Fat – remaining calories from (good) fat.

PUTTING IT ALL TOGETHER

An example; Dave weighs 175lbs., is 35 years old, 6ft and is quite active (runs 1-2 times a week).

- Total calories – 2445 calories

- Carbs – 30 grams / 120 calories

- Protein – 80 grams / 300 calories (using 2.2 g per lb. of body weight)

- Fat – 225 grams / 2025 calories (1778 total calories – (120+300 calories) – 9 calories per gram of fat, hence 1580 calories / 9 = 175 grams of fat required)

Everyone plays by different rules as everyone's body is different; people come in all different shapes and sizes (and metabolisms). The above calculations are a starting point for you to adjust as you become more familiar with how your body is changing.

We are not aiming for perfection, instead we are aiming to get the nutritional inputs to be the *best they can*, without spending weeks tweaking and testing them all down to the last gram.

STEP 3 – MONITORING AND OPTIMIZING

Have We Achieved Ketosis?

Our primary goal is to be in a state of ketosis. How do we know if we are in ketosis? One way to measure is by using ketone testing strips. This measures the concentration of ketones in your system. Ketones are produced by our liver when carbs are restricted. These are transported from the liver to other tissues where they can be reconverted by enzymes in the body to produce energy.

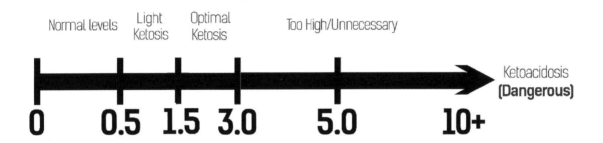

If you do opt for this approach as a guideline, a normal diet will produce ketone levels of under 0.5 mmol/l, however on a ketogenic diet we are aiming for 1.5 – 3.0 mmol/l for the optimal state of ketosis.

Over 5.0mmol/l is unnecessary and over 10.0 is unhealthy as we are at a risk of ketoacidosis. However within the first week as our body is adapting it can be normal to have levels over 3.0 mmol/l.

If testing is not possible or you prefer not to test, then an alternative measure is to go by how you feel:

- Did you go through the 'keto flu'? More energy, increased focus? If not then adjustments may be needed.

- Weight and visual inspection? Have you lost weight? Do you look slimmer? If so, you are likely on the right track.

If you are happy that you are in ketosis then we can move onto the next stage, otherwise try reducing your carb intake by 5g a day and review after one more week. If you wanted to eat more carbs, then you can try increasing your carb intake by 5g a day and see if you are still in ketosis after another week.

'If you cannot measure it, you cannot improve it.'

William Thompson - Physicist

MONITORING

The first four weeks allows us to adjust to the diet, both psychologically and physically. By recording these changes (along with our nutritional intake), it allows us to adjust the diet to our needs. I would recommend recording the below for the first four weeks:

- Weight at the beginning of week 1, end of week 2 and end of week 4. Record your weight under the same conditions each time (ideally first thing in the morning before food).

- Calories – this includes total number of calories as well as the breakdown of fats, proteins and carbs. An app such as MyFitnessPal will do this for you.

- Pictures of yourself (front and side on) at the beginning of week 1, end of week 2 and end of week 4.

- How your feel on a daily basis both physically and emotionally. A simple journal will suffice or a mood tracking app.

- Ketone levels daily. I would recommend some cheap ketone sticks from Amazon.

- Activity levels – How much exercise have you done, and number of estimated calories burnt (again, MyFitnessPal is great for this).

At the end of four weeks, review the data and look back at the changes you have made. You can then start to optimize our diet according to the results.

OPTIMIZING

If you are satisfied that you have reached ketosis, then you know how many grams of carbs you need per day. This is now fixed and **does not change**!

You should also have a good idea of the amount of protein you require (based on your activity level). Again, this becomes fixed (within reason).

With our carb and protein intake being fixed, the only adjustments you need to make are calories coming from fat.

The next step is to begin adjusting the diet so you are making progress towards your goals. Most people have one of two goals, to be healthier or to lose fat. That is to remain the weight they currently are or to lose weight (in the form of fat).

If your goal is fat loss, then it is likely you will begin to make progress in the early stages of the diet. At some point you will likely plateau (weight, measurements do not change much), which is when we need to change the total calorie intake. Adjust the total number of calories by 200 per day across 2-3 weeks and then review your key figures (weight, pictures, body fat %, how you feel). If these are improving then stay on the new total numbers of calories.

Only adjust the calories coming from fat, leaving the intake of carbs and protein the same (assuming you are happy with them).

Once you reach a point you are happy with your weight, you will then attempt to maintain your current weight. Continue to consume the total number of calories you require to maintain your current weight.

Depending on your circumstances, you will likely reach a weight you are happy with between 2-6 months. After this period you will likely over the whole "diet" thing; counting calories, watching what you want stringently etc. I believe that once you have reached your maintenance weight, you can move to a more relaxed way of eating, which is covered in the next section.

Caution – Avoid severely limiting your calorie intake. Only reduce your calorie intake by 200 - 400 a week and never reduce your total calorie intake below 1200 for a woman and 1400 for a man.

PART III – ADAPTING THE DIET TO YOUR LIFE

IT'S ALL A LEARNING CURVE

How do you stop counting calories forever? You make your decisions about food intuitive. How do you do this? Experience, learning, time, and patience.

Consider when you learned to drive a car. At first you had to use a lot of willpower and effort, consciously thinking and acting. But now...you almost drive instinctively and it is likely you do not drive like you were taught. You have taken what they taught you and adapted it to your personality (e.g. you may drive slightly faster than you were taught, you may turn corners one handed). The same process happens when starting a diet.

At the beginning of a diet, you are learning. It takes a lot of willpower and discipline. However, as time goes by, you learn a lot more about the diet and begin to adapt it to your lifestyle. In addition, the amount of discipline and willpower needed decreases. Let's explore what this journey looks like.

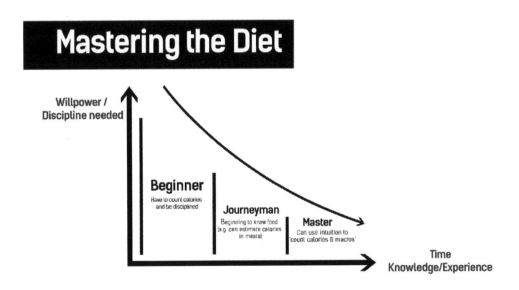

RULES VS PRINCIPLES

I know some people love writing every calorie down, it gives a real sense of reward that they have stuck to their diets religiously. Whereas I know others (myself included) who find that to be a massive chore and would prefer just to eat within tolerable margins of error. This is where the principles versus rules comes in.

Attempting the diet by 'rules' entails recording all your food, how many calories and the types of foods (carbs/protein/ fat) and monitoring these on a regular basis.

'Principle' based dieting is adhering to certain guidelines while being tolerant of adaptations that may be required *(no more counting calories!).* This comes from experience, knowing roughly how many carbs are in each food, and how to stay near the carb limit while staying within the total number of recommended calories.

I prefer principle based eating. I know that I am within 80% of my total calories and carb intake, which is *good enough* to keep me healthy and happy.

The key question is what is "good enough"? Are you preparing for a wedding/holiday where you feel you have to be in your "best" condition, or are you just looking to be healthy and are happy with a few tolerances?

I would always recommend people begin with rules as only experience can provide you with the "principles" that you need. For example, how do you know how many calories are in a bit of cheese unless you have been recording it (rules based) for a few weeks? I would recommended using a rules based approach for about 3-4 weeks and then moving to onto principles based. This will provide you with a strong fundamental knowledge and also confidence to follow your diet.

"80% is good enough in 80% of situations, 80% of the time."

Dan Sullivan – 80% Approach

80% APPROACH – NO MORE COUNTING CALORIES

If the rule based method is working well for you (it has become habitual and is natural to you now), I would suggest continuing with it. If it isn't broken then why fix it?

However if you would like a more relaxed variation of the diet then this may be for you. By now, you should have two things:

- An optimized diet plan, where you know how many carbs and total calories you need to achieve your goals (whether this goal is simply to maintain weight and be healthy or lose weight).

- A good grasp of the types of foods and their calorie content.

With the two above bits of knowledge, you can now operate within certain tolerances. However the general principles of the ketogenic diet still need to be adhered to:

- Low enough carbs to remain in ketosis (likely 30-50 grams)
- Adequate protein
- Enough fats to make up the rest of the total calorie count
- Eating enough calories overall

From this you can create your own guidelines which fit in with you lifestyle.

Unless you are competing in a sport, calorie counting will be excessive and unsustainable in everyday life. I recommend using the 80% Approach which states you can have a 20% margin of error with your nutrition:

- **Total calories** – Allowing a 20% variance in daily calorie intake.
  - If you require 2000, then eat between 1600 – 2400 calories.

- **Eating clean foods** - 80% of the calories are "clean" – the remaining 20% are a cheat meal (usually chocolate in my case).
- **Calories from carbs** – Allowing a 20% variance compared to my usual carb intake.

The above must be used with your own judgment though. Eating 120% of everything (20% more calories, 20% from junk food, 20% more carbs) every day for a month is not recommended.

From a physical and psychological point of view, I recommend continuing to measure yourself every 2 – 4 weeks, in terms of body measurements, weight, and photos. Psychologically this retains a sense of accountability to yourself (e.g. you know the weigh-in is next week so you will maintain some discipline). It will also tell you whether your principles are working or not.

The Next Level – Creating Your Own Rules

You can then take this one step further and develop your own principles based on your knowledge of food and how your body works. This is only recommended once you have followed the diet for at least six months.

This will involve moving away from calories and toward food being units (which you get to make up!).

For example, my principles are on a daily basis:

- Carbs – below are my either/or principles for any one day (e.g. beans or quinoa)

  - Eating as many beans as I like
  - No more than a cup of a grain (mostly quinoa)
  - No more than 1 slice of bread

- Protein

  - At least one piece of meat a day
  - At least one piece of fish a day
  - At least one protein shake a day

- Fats – This is more from a feeling. I will eat three meals a day, and I eat enough just to feel satiated. I have learned over time how big my portions should be for me to feel satiated at the end of every meal.

PART IV - MAKING A GOOD START

"The secret to success is learning how to use pain and pleasure, instead of having pain and pleasure use you."

Tony Robbins - Self-development guru

WHY MOST DIETS FAIL & HOW TO KEEP ON TRACK

I am a big fan of Tony Robbins (self-development guru). One of his most powerful ideas is that there are two forces which motivate people: a desire to **avoid pain** and a desire to **gain pleasure**. These, in turn, affect our beliefs which impact our behavior.

For example, I have a belief that doing the household chores is boring. The pain of **not** doing the household chores (a dirty house), is **more painful** than the pain of **doing it** (getting all dirty and smelling like bleach for two hours).

The same with pleasure; the pleasure of **not** doing the household chores (having more free time to have coffee and hang out with friends) is **greater** than the pleasure of doing the chores (having a clean house).

If I have this belief system, am I likely to ever clean the house? Only when the pain of **not** doing it becomes more painful than doing it, e.g. when my mum arrives and complains for 4 straight hours about how dirty it is (true pain to me).

Whereas my partner is different. He loves household chores and takes massive pride in doing so. The pain of not doing the chores (visitors thinking he is slothful) is greater than **not** doing it. He also takes pleasure from doing it (pride that his "castle" is clean and he can listen to an audiobook at the same time).

This same principle is why most diets fail, people start with good intentions, knowing that in the long-run they will lose weight (avoiding pain) and feel healthier (moving towards pleasure), but the pain of continuing the diet (e.g. not being able to eat out with friends) is greater than sticking to the diet. Also, there is often no pleasure in the diet either (it is seen as much more pleasurable to just eat cake than a boring salad).

Generally people fail to start or maintain diets because:

- It is a "diet" – Diets have become synonymous with pain.

- They are for martyrs – Only eating cabbage for a month? That definitely sounds like pain!

- Inconsistent with lifestyle – Some diets are hard work, requiring a massive lifestyle change which is seen as a lot of work (pain) hence it is easier not to change.

For me, a diet should be pleasurable and the pain of doing them should be less than not doing them. Some criteria that I look for:

- Fits in easily with my lifestyle – It does not require a massive change outside of my current lifestyle.

- It should be a "lifestyle" not a "diet" – It is a long term solution, not a temporary fix (hence the well-known concept of yoyo dieting).

- The food is pleasurable – I want to look forward to eating my food.

- It is easy – I am not a chef, and want to be able to make simple delicious food quickly.

- The benefits of the diet are aligned with my goals – What are your goals and is this type of diet right for you?

The ketogenic guide and the recipes in this book aim to fulfill all of these requirements:

- Fits in with my lifestyle – I do not need to change my eating patterns massively (I can still eat breakfast, lunch and dinner).

- Is aimed toward long term health and is not a crash diet.

- Food is pleasurable – I associate "fat" food with being delicious. I am able to eat steak, cheese and a whole host of other great foods more often.

- It is easy – there are 100 recipes in this book all of which are easy and can be made within 20 minutes. Also the "80% principle" (explained later) helps too.

- Aligned with my goals – I want to feel better on the inside and lose fat, these are some of the key benefits of ketogenic diets.

PREPARING FOR A POSITIVE START

Before beginning the diet, below is a good primer on what to expect and some helpful tips for when you start out.

Preparations Before Starting

Understand your body is adapting in the first two weeks - You may feel slightly low on energy as your body adapts to using different energy sources. Simply recognize it for what it is (your body is adapting), and know it is only temporary. Ultimately you will reap the benefits.

Clear out the cupboard in advance – If you are like me, if it is in the cupboard, then it gets eaten. Clear out the cupboard of anything you will not be eating on the diet (mostly processed carbs), thus removing the temptation.

Get a calorie counter – Such as the MyFitnessPal app. While the idea of calorie counting turns a lot of people off, they provide the fundamental knowledge of how many calories/carbs are in different types of foods. This allows you to move from calorie counting to a "principle based" diet in the future (more on that later).

Don't be obsessed with weighing yourself – Your weight can vary as much as 4 lbs. on any given day. While I recommend tracking weight (every two weeks at first then monthly), weighing yourself every day is counterproductive. Focus instead on the general health benefits.

Think ahead of social situations – It is all too easy to get caught up in social situations and revert to old habits. Instead think ahead of time, for example, bring your own snacks to work rather than eating the biscuits everyone else is having.

Tip – *Do not keep it a secret – Let your friends and family know what you are doing. People tend to be more understanding and supportive if they are aware you are working towards a change in lifestyle.*

Plan ahead and create a routine– Particularly in the first few weeks. You are attempting to establish new habits, which requires a conscious effort to establish and to not fall back into old habits. Plan your meals the week/day before, otherwise it is too easy to grab a chocolate bar "just this one time" because you are in a hurry.

Monitor your ketone levels – Not compulsory, but recommended. I would suggest some cheap ketone test strips from Amazon (more on their use later).

General Eating Principles to Remember

A calorie is not just a calorie – It may sound obvious but not all fats or proteins were created equally, focus on good quality fats.

Eat enough calories – This is not a low calorie diet, nor is it an excuse to eat as many hamburgers as you want. Follow the guidelines below and ensure you are getting the right amount of calories

Eat your vegetables – It can be very easy to focus on the fat sources and neglect a balanced diet. Try to have at least one cup of vegetables a day.

If you really have to drink alcohol then try to go for low carb options. Spirits with low carb mixers are probably the best option or dry white wines (obviously in moderation). Avoid any alcoholic drinks with added sugar (e.g. Bacardi Breezer).

Drink plenty of water – It goes without saying!

Try to eat natural as much as possible – While there have been many studies for and against the benefits of organic food, it comes down to personal preference. I would suggest trying it for 2-3 weeks and see if you feel a difference.

Eat clean as much as possible – Try to eat foods which are still in their natural state, e.g. fresh fruit (rather than frozen), fresh beef (rather than processed into something else), chocolate (if you have to have it) in as raw a format you can (rather than processed and additives/sugar added etc.).

FINAL NOTES

Adjusting and customizing the recipes

These recipes have been created to be:

1. Easy to make

2. Delicious

3. Easy to find ingredients

However, there is not a one size fits all recipe, everyone has different tastes, some have allergies and not everyone will be able to get all of the ingredients. Consider the recipes as a guideline which you can then customize to your own taste or to what you have in the house.

- Do not like cilantro? Consider switching it with parsley.. or leave it out entirely.

- Do not have any pink rock salt in the house? Just use some normal table salt instead.

- Do not like venison? Try beef instead.

- Prefer your eggs a bit runnier? Cook them for slightly less time.

- Do not want to cook 4 servings? Simply halve the ingredients and only cook 2.

- Do not have a spiralizer? Just cut into strip or just use a peeler.

I have included some suggestions throughout for alternatives, but could not list every single one. Only you know what your preferences are, so have some fun with it and play around with different ingredients and recipes.

Thank you

Whether you are new to ketogenic diets or have been exploring this for a while, I hope you have found this guide useful and will take up the ideas to create a healthier and more balanced lifestyle for yourself.

I am always looking to improve my works and to help me create the best book I can, I would like to hear your honest feedback and what you found most useful and what could be improved.

I would be most appreciative if you would leave an honest review of this book on Amazon.

Please visit the link below to leave an honest review:

http://geni.us/Keto100review

And just another quick reminder to download the Quick Start Guide and 7 Day Meal Planner to help make the first week as easy as possible.

Download your copy from the link - http://geni.us/keto100land

Once again, thank you for downloading and good luck.

Elizabeth Jane

YOU MAY ALSO LIKE...

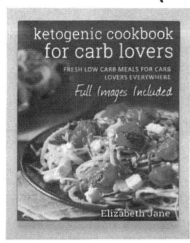

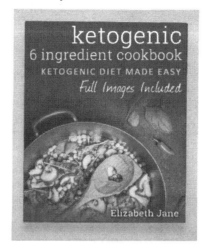

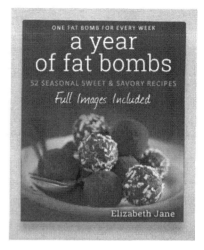

If you miss your favorite carbohydrate dishes on a low carb diet, then this book is for you.

- Continue to burn fat whilst eating your favorite sandwiches, traditional lasagna and keto pizza.

- Please visit the below link to get your copy: http://geni.us/CarbLover

I created this book by listening to your feedback.

You wanted:

- Quicker and easier meals
- All recipes with 6 ingredients or less
- All made in under 20 minutes
- Please visit the below link to get your http://geni.us/6ingketo

My most recent book is perhaps my most challenging and creative yet, a year's worth of fat bombs.

The recipes are:

- Seasonal – Created according to the season, both in taste and ingredient availability.

- Not just sweet – Includes savory fat bombs too.

- Obviously...all delicious.

Please visit the below link to get your copy: http://geni.us/KetoFatBomb

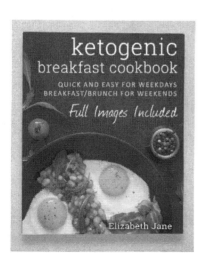

Breakfast is the most important keto meal of the day! This book was created to:

- Help you make great quick and easy meals during the week
- Have delicious brunch meals on the weekend

Please visit the below link to get your http://geni.us/Ketobreakfast

PART V - RECIPES

THYME AND PAPRIKA SHRIMP

Preparation time: 10 minutes
Cooking time: 10 minutes

Serves: 3

1 pound fresh shrimp (peeled and deveined)
5 sprigs fresh thyme (only leaves)
2 tablespoons olive oil
1 teaspoon paprika
Black pepper to taste
Salt to taste

NUTRITIONAL INFO (PER SERVING)

Total Carbohydrates: 6g
Dietary Fiber: 2g
Net Carbs: 4g
Protein: 35g
Total Fat: 12g
Calories: 275

DIRECTIONS:

1. Mix the shrimp, thyme and paprika together in a mixing bowl and season to taste with black pepper and salt. Mix well to ensure the shrimp has an even coating of all ingredients.

2. Heat up the olive oil in a large frying pan over high heat. Wait for the oil to get hot, then add the shrimp. Let the shrimp cook, stirring often, for about 6 minutes, until the shrimp is opaque and cooked through.

3. Remove the frying pan from the heat. Divide the shrimp between three plates and serve warm. Decorate with fresh thyme sprigs on top and sprinkle paprika.

SALMON STIR FRY WITH BROCCOLI AND PEAS

Preparation time: 10 minutes **Serves:** 6
Cooking time: 15 minutes

1 pound fresh broccoli (cut into florets)
1 ½ pounds fresh salmon fillets (cut into cubes)
1 tablespoon olive oil
3 garlic cloves (minced)
2 medium onions (halved and thinly sliced)
¼ pound frozen peas
1 tablespoon sesame seeds
2 tablespoons soy sauce
1 tablespoon chopped parsley
1 teaspoon toasted sesame oil

NUTRITIONAL INFO (PER SERVING)

Total Carbohydrates: 12g
Dietary Fiber: 4g
Net Carbs: 8g
Protein: 26g
Total Fat: 11g
Calories: 240

DIRECTIONS:

1. Add the olive oil to a wok over high heat. Once the oil is hot, add the garlic and stir constantly for about 20 seconds. Add the salmon and cook until it changes color.

2. Add onion, broccoli and peas to the wok and stir occasionally for 5 minutes or until the vegetables are soft.

3. Add the soy sauce, sesame oil and chopped parsley. Stir these ingredients in and then gently toss to coat before removing the wok from the heat.

4. Divide between six plates, sprinkle extra parsley and sesame seeds on top of each portion and add a lemon wedge right before serving (optional).

ASIAN TUNA WITH PARSLEY

Preparation time: 5 minutes
Cooking time: 15 minutes

Serves: 2

3 tablespoons coconut oil

2 cloves garlic (crushed)

½ pound fresh tuna fillets (cut into slices)

5 tablespoons coconut milk

1 tablespoon fish sauce

Ground black pepper to taste

Salt to taste

Small bunch fresh parsley (chopped)

NUTRITIONAL INFO (PER SERVING)

Total Carbohydrates: 5g
Dietary Fiber: 2g
Net Carbs: 4g
Protein: 32g
Total Fat: 39g
Calories: 490

DIRECTIONS:

1. Add coconut oil to a skillet or frying pan over a medium heat. Once the oil is hot, add crushed garlic and sauté for about 2 minutes, until soft.

2. Add the tuna slices and sauté for about 3 minutes, until the tuna is cooked.

3. Stirring carefully, add the coconut milk, fish sauce, ground black pepper and salt. Sauté for about 1 minute.

4. Divide the tuna between 2 plates or set out on a serving dish. Sprinkle chopped parsley.

5. Pour any remaining liquid from the skillet over the shrimp and sprinkle with chopped cilantro before serving.

CUCUMBER NOODLES WITH SHRIMP

Preparation time: 10 minutes
Cooking time: 15 minutes

Serves: 5

2 cucumbers (preferably seedless)
½ pound fresh shrimp (peeled and deveined)
1 tablespoon Thai red curry paste
½ scallion or spring onion (chopped)
2 garlic cloves (finely chopped)
1 ounce ginger (finely chopped)
1 tablespoon soy sauce
1 tablespoon olive oil
½ green chili (finely chopped)
½ bunch cilantro (finely chopped)
1 tablespoon chopped peanuts to decorate

NUTRITIONAL INFO (PER SERVING)

Total Carbohydrates: 11g
Dietary Fiber: 2g
Net Carbs: 9g
Protein: 13g
Total Fat: 6g
Calories: 145

DIRECTIONS:

1. Use a spiralizer, mandolin or vegetable peeler to turn the cucumbers into spaghetti or tagliatelle noodles. Place the noodles in a small bowl and set aside.

2. Heat the olive oil over a medium heat and sauté the scallion, garlic, ginger and chili for about 2 minutes.

3. Stir in the curry paste, soy sauce and half the cilantro. Sauté for another 2 minutes.

4. Add the shrimp and cover evenly in the sauce. Cook for about 8 minutes.

5. Divide the noodles between 2 plates and then carefully add the shrimp to each plate. Decorate with chopped peanuts.

6. Sprinkle with remaining cilantro. Serve right away.

BAKED SEA BASS WITH MUSTARD SAUCE

Preparation time: 15 minutes (plus 2 hours in fridge)

Cooking time: 25 minutes
Serves: 5

For the Sea Bass

- 5 tablespoons lemon juice
- 2 tablespoons olive oil
- 4 tablespoons fresh oregano (chopped)
- Salt to taste
- Freshly ground black pepper to taste
- 1 ½ pounds sea bass fillets

For the mustard sauce

- 2 tablespoons Dijon mustard
- 3 ounces fat-free sour cream
- 1 teaspoon olive oil
- 2 tablespoons fresh oregano (chopped)
- Pinch of brown sugar
- Salt to taste
- Freshly ground black pepper to taste

NUTRITIONAL INFO (PER SERVING)

Total Carbohydrates: 7g
Dietary Fiber: 3g
Net Carbs: 5g
Protein: 33g
Total Fat: 11g
Calories: 265

DIRECTIONS:

1. Add the lemon juice, olive oil, chopped oregano, salt and ground black pepper to a medium bowl and mix until well combined.

2. Place the sea bass fillets into a baking dish and pour the marinade over them. Turn the fillets over to ensure each fillet is well covered in the juice. Cover the baking dish with a lid or plastic wrap and refrigerate for 2 hours to allow the sea bass to marinate.

3. To make the mustard sauce, add the Dijon mustard to a bowl and then slowly stir in the olive oil. Next, add the sour cream, pinch of brown sugar, oregano, salt and

ground black pepper, continuing to mix as you add each ingredient. Cover and refrigerate for 2 hours.

4. Take the sea bass out of the fridge and wrap in a loose parcel using aluminum foil, ensuring the sauce cannot run out of the sides. Bake in preheated oven (400°F) for 20 minutes, until the fish is cooked through.

5. Unwrap the fish and place each fillet on a serving plate. Cover with the mustard sauce and serve immediately.

CREAMY SALMON WITH EGGPLANT

Preparation time: 15 minutes
Cooking time: 30 minutes

Serves: 5

For the Sauce:

- 5 ounces sour cream
- 1 teaspoon paprika
- 1 teaspoon fresh parsley (chopped)
- Salt to taste

For the Salmon:

- 1 pound fresh salmon fillets
- Salt to taste
- Black pepper to taste
- Fresh oregano (chopped) to taste

For the eggplant:

- 2 large eggplants (cut into strips)
- Salt to taste
- Black pepper to taste

NUTRITIONAL INFO (PER SERVING)

Total Carbohydrates: 13g
Dietary Fiber: 5g
Net Carbs: 8g
Protein: 20g
Total Fat: 6g
Calories: 186

DIRECTIONS:
----

1. To make the sauce, add the paprika and a pinch of salt in a bowl and gradually whisk in the sour cream to achieve a smooth consistency. Stir in the parsley. Refrigerate.

2. Place the salmon and the eggplant strips into a greased baking dish. Season with salt, pepper and oregano.

3. Preheat the oven to 450°F. Cover the dish with aluminum foil and place it in the center of the oven and bake for about 20 minutes. Remove the aluminum foil and bake for 10 minutes more.

4. Take the dish out of the oven and gently place the salmon fillets and the eggplant strips on a serving plate.

5. Pour the sauce over the top. Add salt to taste and garnish with fresh oregano (optional).

GINGER COD WITH ZUCCHINI NOODLES

Preparation time: 20 minutes   **Serves:** 4
Cooking time: 10 minutes
Marinating time: 40 minutes (optional)

3 large zucchini, spiralized (alternatively, use a julienne peeler or slice into thin strips)

1 ½ pounds fresh cod fillets

2 inches fresh ginger (finely chopped)

3 tablespoons soy sauce

2 tablespoons rice vinegar

1 green onion (chopped)

1 garlic clove (minced)

1 cup vegetable broth

1 bunch fresh parsley (finely chopped)

NUTRITIONAL INFO (PER SERVING)

Total Carbohydrates: 13g
Dietary Fiber: 3g
Net Carbs: 10g
Protein: 27g
Total Fat: 2g
Calories: 175

DIRECTIONS:
----

1. Use a spiralizer, mandolin, julienne or vegetable peeler to turn the zucchini into noodles.

2. Combine the chopped ginger, garlic, soy sauce, vegetable broth, green onions and vinegar in a medium bowl.

3. Chop the cod fillets into strips and put them in the bowl with the mixture. Turn the strips over to ensure they are fully coated in the mixture and let them marinate for 40 minutes.

4. Heat a large nonstick frying pan over a medium heat, add some olive oil and cook the cod for about 4 minutes on each side. Add the marinade to the pan, bring to a boil and then immediately remove from the heat.

5. Divide the noodles into four portions, add the cod on top and pour the sauce over the fish. Sprinkle chopped parsley on top and serve right away.

SPINACH SALAD WITH SALMON, STRAWBERRIES AND WALNUTS

Preparation time: 10 minutes
Cooking time: 20 minutes

Serves: 5

Salad

- 5 ounces baby spinach leaves
- 2 ripe avocados (chopped)
- 8 ripe strawberries (chopped)
- 5 ounces cherry tomatoes (halved)
- 2 ounces walnuts (chopped)
- 1 pound fresh salmon fillets
- 1 teaspoon olive oil

Vinaigrette

- 2 tablespoons fresh lemon juice
- 6 tablespoons olive oil
- 1 teaspoon Dijon mustard
- 1 pinch cayenne pepper

NUTRITIONAL INFO (PER SERVING)

Total Carbohydrates: 12g
Dietary Fiber: 8g
Net Carbs: 5g
Protein: 23g
Total Fat: 46g
Calories: 526

DIRECTIONS:

1. Preheat the oven to 400°F.

2. Heat a cast iron or oven-proof pan over a medium-high heat and add the olive oil once the pan is hot.

3. Place the salmon in the pan skin-side down and cook the fillets for about 4 minutes.

4. Transfer the pan to the middle shelf in the oven and continue cooking for about 4 minutes (depending on the thickness) until cooked through.

5. Add the spinach, chopped avocado, strawberries, cherry tomatoes and walnuts to a large bowl.

6. Mix the freshly squeezed lemon juice with the Dijon mustard in another small bowl and whisk. Continue to whisk while gradually adding the olive oil. Once the vinaigrette is well combined, season it with cayenne pepper.

7. Divide the salad between two plates or bowls, add the salmon on top of each serving and then drizzle the vinaigrette over the top. Serve right away!

TUNA WITH TOMATOES AND PARSLEY

Preparation time: 5 minutes
Cooking time: 20 minutes

Serves: 4

10 ounces cherry tomatoes
2 tablespoons olive oil
Salt to taste
Ground black pepper to taste
1 ½ pounds fresh tuna fillets (cut into cubes)
2 teaspoons ground turmeric
1 bunch fresh parsley (chopped)

NUTRITIONAL INFO (PER SERVING)

Total Carbohydrates: 4g
Dietary Fiber: 2g
Net Carbs: 3g
Protein: 41g
Total Fat: 20g
Calories: 360

DIRECTIONS:

1. Preheat the oven to 400°F.

2. Add the tomatoes, olive oil, salt, and black pepper to a bowl and mix well. Pour this mixture into a baking tray and spread it out evenly.

3. Place the tuna on top of the tomato mixture. Coat the tuna with the oil from the baking tray using a pastry brush or the back of a spoon. Then, sprinkle turmeric, more salt and ground black pepper over the top of the tuna.

4. Roast the fish in the oven for about 15 minutes or until the tuna flakes easily when tested with a fork.

5. Garnish with chopped parsley.

STEAMED COD

Preparation time: 15 minutes
Cooking time: 20 minutes

Serves: 4

2 tablespoons olive oil
3 cloves garlic (chopped)
4 tablespoons fresh thyme (chopped)
½ cup white wine
1 cup vegetable broth
3 tablespoons butter
1 ½ pounds cod fillets (cut into large pieces)
Ground black pepper to taste
Fresh thyme (for garnish)

NUTRITIONAL INFO (PER SERVING)

Total Carbohydrates: 4g
Dietary Fiber: 1g
Net Carbs: 3g
Protein: 36g
Total Fat: 18g
Calories: 340

DIRECTIONS:

1. Add the olive oil to a large pot over high heat. Once the oil is hot, add the garlic and sauté for about 2 minutes. Add the chopped thyme, wine, broth and butter. Mix gently and bring it to a boil.

2. Once it is boiling, add the cod fillets and cover the pot with a lid. Reduce the heat and cook for 5 minutes, stirring occasionally.

3. Share the fish equally between 4 serving bowls.

4. Season the cod with salt and pepper and pour the hot broth over the top.

5. Garnish with fresh thyme.

TRUFFLE TUNA STEAKS

Preparation time: 5 minutes
Cooking time: 15 minutes
Serves: 3

    1 ½ pounds fresh tuna steaks
    2 tablespoons truffle oil
    3 tablespoons olive oil
    2 tablespoons chopped fresh oregano

NUTRITIONAL INFO (PER SERVING)

Total Carbohydrates: 1g
Dietary Fiber: 1g
Net Carbs: 0g
Protein: 40g
Total Fat: 23g
Calories: 380

DIRECTIONS:

1. Sprinkle the truffle oil over both sides of the tuna steaks, distributing it evenly.

2. Add the olive oil to a large frying pan over high heat.

3. Once the oil is hot, add the tuna steaks and cook for about 4 minutes on each side. Serve right away!

SALMON, ALMONDS AND FENNEL SALAD

Preparation time: 10 minutes   **Serves:** 5
Cooking time: 0 minutes

Zest of a lemon

2 tablespoons lemon juice

1 teaspoon curry powder

3 tablespoons olive oil

4 tablespoons fresh oregano (chopped)

1 bunch of fresh parsley (chopped)

1 small fennel bulb (thinly shaved with a peeler)

1 cucumber (cut into pieces)

10 ounces canned salmon (drained and flaked)

2 ounces sliced almonds

Salt to taste

Black pepper to taste

NUTRITIONAL INFO (PER SERVING)

Total Carbohydrates: 11g
Dietary Fiber: 5g
Net Carbs: 6g
Protein: 15g
Total Fat: 18g
Calories: 254

DIRECTIONS:
----

1. In a small bowl, combine the lemon zest, lemon juice, curry, olive oil, a pinch of salt and ground black pepper together, mix well.

2. In a medium bowl, add the chopped oregano and parsley, followed by the fennel, cucumber and salmon. Pour in the lemon dressing. Mix well.

3. Divide the salad between two serving plates and sprinkle sliced almonds over the top. Enjoy!

SALMON STEAKS, ITALIAN-STYLE

Preparation time: 10 minutes
(plus 2 hours in fridge)

Cooking time: 20 minutes
Serves: 6

5 tablespoons fresh basil

6 garlic cloves (minced)

1 teaspoon ground paprika

½ pound fresh tomatoes (chopped)

5 tablespoons olive oil

2 pounds fresh salmon fillets

Salt to taste

Black pepper to taste

NUTRITIONAL INFO (PER SERVING)

Total Carbohydrates: 3g
Dietary Fiber: 1g
Net Carbs: 2g
Protein: 30g
Total Fat: 21g
Calories: 310

DIRECTIONS:

1. Use a blender or food processor to mix the fresh basil, garlic and paprika. Slowly add the olive oil while the blender or food processor is running (carefully). Blend until you have a smooth sauce.

2. Put the salmon fillets in a large bowl and cover with about half of the sauce. Cover the bowl with plastic wrap and refrigerate for 2 hours.

3. Take the salmon fillets out of the bowl and season with salt and black pepper. Grill the salmon fillets for about 3 minutes on each side.

4. Place each of the salmon fillets on a serving plate, top with chopped tomatoes and drizzle with the remaining sauce.

SALMON MOZZARELLA SALAD

Preparation time: 15 minutes   **Serves:** 4
Cooking time: 0 minutes

½ pound cherry tomatoes (halved)
4 ounces fresh mozzarella (cut into small cubes)
1 cucumber (chopped)
4 tablespoons fresh thyme (chopped)
10 ounces canned salmon (drained)
1 tablespoon rice vinegar
3 tablespoons olive oil
Salt to taste
Black pepper to taste

NUTRITIONAL INFO (PER SERVING)

Total Carbohydrates: 8g
Dietary Fiber: 2g
Net Carbs: 6g
Protein: 23g
Total Fat: 20g
Calories: 295

DIRECTIONS:

1. Put the cherry tomatoes in a bowl, then add the chopped cucumber, fresh thyme and salmon. Stir and then add the mozzarella to the bowl.

2. Stir in the vinegar and olive oil, season with salt and black pepper. Toss the salad gently in the bowl before serving. Serve right away!

SHRIMP AND LEMON NOODLES

Preparation time: 20 minutes
Cooking time: 10 minutes

Serves: 5

2 cucumbers
3 cups cauliflower (cut into small pieces)
1 small red onion (finely chopped)
3 ounces pitted olives (halved)
1 pound fresh shrimp (peeled and deveined)
1 ½ lemons (juice and zest)
1 tablespoon capers
3 tablespoons olive oil (plus extra for drizzling)
Salt to taste
Black pepper to taste

NUTRITIONAL INFO (PER SERVING)

Total Carbohydrates: 13g
Dietary Fiber: 4g
Net Carbs: 10g
Protein: 23g
Total Fat: 12g
Calories: 272

DIRECTIONS:

1. Spiralize the cucumber (or cut into strips) and place in a bowl.

2. Heat 1 tablespoon of olive oil in a frying pan, add the shrimp and cook until opaque and pink, stirring occasionally.

3. In a separate bowl, combine the cooked shrimp, olives, red onion, capers, lemon zest and juice. Toss gently then add the cauliflower and cucumber noodles. Mix well and ensure a good coating of the mixture on the cauliflower and cucumber.

4. Drizzle the remaining olive oil in the bowl and season with the black pepper. Toss a little more and enjoy!

Citrus Shrimp Pepper Salad

Preparation time: 15 minutes
Cooking time: 10 minutes

Serves: 4

1 yellow bell pepper (sliced)
1 green bell pepper (sliced)
3 large tomatoes (chopped)
1 bunch of fresh parsley (chopped)
1 pound fresh shrimp (peeled and deveined)
1 lemon (juice)
1 tablespoon olive oil
Salt to taste
Pepper to taste

NUTRITIONAL INFO (PER SERVING)

Total Carbohydrates: 12g
Dietary Fiber: 3g
Net Carbs: 9g
Protein: 28g
Total Fat: 12g
Calories: 275

DIRECTIONS:

1. Heat the olive oil in a frying pan, add the shrimp and cook until opaque and pink, stirring occasionally. Set aside.

2. Put the bell peppers in a large bowl. Add the chopped tomatoes and parsley, then squeeze the lemon juice over the top.

3. Add the cooked shrimp and stir or toss gently to mix the salad together. Season with salt and pepper to taste.

4. Divide between two plates or bowls. Garnish with parsley.

TUNA AND MUSHROOM SALAD

Preparation time: 10 minutes
Cooking time: 5 minutes

Serves: 4

½ small onion (thinly sliced)
10 ounces canned tuna (drained and flaked)
½ pound cup fresh white mushrooms (sliced)
½ pound cherry tomatoes (halved)
4 tablespoons olive oil
2 teaspoons Dijon mustard
2 ounces fresh dill (chopped)
Salt to taste
Black pepper to taste

NUTRITIONAL INFO (PER SERVING)

Total Carbohydrates: 13g
Dietary Fiber: 4g
Net Carbs: 10g
Protein: 24g
Total Fat: 21g
Calories: 315

DIRECTIONS:

1. Heat 1 tablespoon of olive oil in a frying pan, add mushrooms and cook for about 4 minutes, stirring occasionally. Set aside.

2. Add the sliced onion, tuna flakes, mushrooms, dill and cherry tomatoes to a large bowl and stir until well combined.

3. In a smaller bowl, add remaining olive oil and the Dijon mustard, mix well. Add salt and black pepper to taste.

4. Pour the dressing on top of the tuna mixture and toss well to combine. Serve right away.

Spicy Shrimp and Lettuce Salad

Preparation time: 15 minutes
Cooking time: 10 minutes

Serves: 4

½ onion (thinly sliced)

5 cups lettuce (shredded)

3 tablespoons olive oil

1 red chili (finely chopped)

1 pound cherry tomatoes (halved)

4 tablespoons parmesan (grated)

1 pound fresh shrimp (peeled and deveined)

5 tablespoons chopped spring onions

Salt to taste

Black pepper to taste

NUTRITIONAL INFO (PER SERVING)

Total Carbohydrates: 13g
Dietary Fiber: 4g
Net Carbs: 10g
Protein: 31g
Total Fat: 15g
Calories: 305

DIRECTIONS:

1. Heat a frying pan over a medium heat and add a tablespoon of olive oil. Once hot, sauté the sliced onion until soft. Add the chili and sauté for about 1 minute to bring out the spice. Transfer to a large bowl and set aside.

2. In the same frying pan, add another tablespoon of olive oil. Once hot, sauté the shrimp until opaque and pink.

3. Combine the cherry tomatoes, lettuce, parmesan, spring onions and shrimp into the bowl with the onions and toss gently.

4. Distribute evenly onto plates and drizzle the remaining olive oil. Add salt and pepper to taste.

WATERCRESS SALMON SALAD WITH OLIVES

Preparation time: 15 minutes   **Serves:** 3
Cooking time: 0 minutes

3 ounces pitted green olives (halved)
10 ounces canned salmon (drained)
1 red onion (finely chopped)
3 cups fresh watercress
3 tablespoons olive oil
1 tablespoon white wine vinegar
2 tablespoons fresh thyme (chopped)
Salt to taste
Black pepper to taste

NUTRITIONAL INFO (PER SERVING)

Total Carbohydrates: 6g
Dietary Fiber: 3g
Net Carbs: 4g
Protein: 20g
Total Fat: 22g
Calories: 300

DIRECTIONS:

1. Add the olives, salmon, watercress, onion and thyme to a large salad bowl and toss gently to combine.

2. Make the dressing in a separate, small bowl by whisking the olive oil and vinegar. Season with salt and pepper. Once combined, pour over the salad.

3. Serve immediately.

Sea Bass Salad with Orange Dressing

Preparation time: 15 minutes
Cooking time: 10 minutes

Serves: 4

1 small spaghetti squash
½ pound fresh sea bass fillets (cut into slices)
1 tablespoon capers (drained)
1 celery stalk (cut into small cubes)
6 ounces cherry tomatoes (halved)
3 tablespoons orange juice
1 tablespoon orange zest
4 tablespoons olive oil
5 cups rocket leaves
4 tablespoons fresh basil (chopped)
Salt to taste
Black pepper to taste

NUTRITIONAL INFO (PER SERVING)

Total Carbohydrates: 8g
Dietary Fiber: 2g
Net Carbs: 7g
Protein: 15g
Total Fat: 16g
Calories: 230

DIRECTIONS:

1. Preheat the oven to 375°F. Slice the squash in half lengthwise then use a spoon to scrape out the seeds. Coat the inside of each half with 1 tablespoon of olive oil and place on a baking sheet. Cover with aluminum foil and place in the oven for about 45 minutes. At this point, you should easily be able to pierce the squash. Use a fork to gently peel the inside flesh into strands. Put the strands into a large bowl and discard the skin.

2. Heat a frying pan over a medium heat and add a tablespoon of olive oil. Once hot, sauté the sliced sea bass until golden brown. Set aside.

3. Add the capers, cooked sea bass, celery, orange zest and cherry tomatoes to the bowl with the spaghetti squash. Toss around gently to mix well. Drizzle the orange juice and the remaining olive oil and toss gently. Season with salt and pepper to taste.

4. Serve with rocket leaves and garnish with fresh basil.

PAN-SEARED SALMON FILLETS

Preparation time: 10 minutes
Cooking time: 15 minutes

Serves: 2

1 pound fresh salmon fillets
Himalayan sea salt to taste
Ground pepper to taste
1 tablespoon butter
3 tablespoons olive oil
1 teaspoon Dijon mustard
1 tablespoon fresh thyme (chopped)

NUTRITIONAL INFO (PER SERVING)
- - - - - - - - - - - - - - - - - - -
Total Carbohydrates: 2g
Dietary Fiber: 1g
Net Carbs: 1g
Protein: 45g
Total Fat: 41g
Calories: 538

DIRECTIONS:
- -

1. Sprinkle the salmon fillets with salt and pepper.

2. In a small bowl, mix 2 tablespoons of olive oil, thyme and the Dijon mustard. Set aside.

3. Melt the butter and 1 tablespoon of olive oil over medium heat in a frying pan.

4. Carefully place the salmon fillets in the frying pan and cook for about 3 minutes per side, or to desired level of doneness.

5. Drizzle the mustard sauce over the fillets. Serve right away.

TUNA AND DILL CREAMY SAUCE

Preparation time: 15 minutes
Cooking time: 15 minutes

Serves: 3

5 ounces broccoli florets (chopped)
5 ounces cherry tomatoes (halved)
3 ounces fresh dill (chopped)
20 ounces canned tuna (drained)
Zest and juice of 1 lemon
4 tablespoons olive oil
2 tablespoons sour cream
Salt to taste
Black pepper to taste

NUTRITIONAL INFO (PER SERVING)

Total Carbohydrates: 13g
Dietary Fiber: 4g
Net Carbs: 10g
Protein: 34g
Total Fat: 22g
Calories: 375

DIRECTIONS:
----

1. Bring a large pot of water to a boil. Blanch the broccoli for about 4 minutes. Set aside four tablespoons of the cooking water before draining and immediately place broccoli in ice water to stop cooking.

2. Add the fresh dill, lemon zest, lemon juice, the cup of cooking water and olive oil to a food processor and process to create a smooth pesto.

3. Heat a skillet or frying pan over medium heat. Add the pesto from the food processor, the tuna, the cherry tomatoes and the sour cream. Stir gently and add the blanched broccoli. Season with salt and pepper to taste.

4. Once hot, remove from heat and serve.

PEAR TUNA SALAD

Preparation time: 10 minutes
Cooking time: 0 minutes

Serves: 5

4 tablespoons celery (chopped)
10 ounces canned tuna (drained)
6 cups rocket leaves
1 pear (cut into small cubes)
1 pinch of ground turmeric
4 ounces mayonnaise

NUTRITIONAL INFO (PER SERVING)

Total Carbohydrates: 11g
Dietary Fiber: 2g
Net Carbs: 10g
Protein: 16g
Total Fat: 13g
Calories: 217

DIRECTIONS:

1. Put the drained tuna in a large bowl and mash with a fork to break up any large chunks. Add the chopped celery and pear, stir well to combine.

2. Add the turmeric, rocket leaves and mayonnaise and mix well until all of the tuna, pear and celery are coated.

3. Serve immediately or refrigerate up to 2 hours.

POACHED SALMON OVER SPINACH SALAD

Preparation time: 10 minutes
Cooking time: 20 minutes

Serves: 5

1 ½ pounds fresh salmon fillets

1 small red onion (finely sliced)

5 tablespoons fresh oregano (chopped)

5 tablespoons fresh parsley (chopped)

1 teaspoon mustard seeds

½ cup olive oil

Salt to taste

Ground black pepper to taste

6 ounces baby spinach leaves

1 tablespoon rice vinegar

1 cup water

NUTRITIONAL INFO (PER SERVING)

Total Carbohydrates: 6g

Dietary Fiber: 3g

Net Carbs: 3g

Protein: 28g

Total Fat: 43g

Calories: 500

DIRECTIONS:

1. Place a large frying pan over a low heat and add ¼ cup of the olive oil. Add the sliced onion, oregano, parsley, mustard seeds, salt, ground black pepper and 1 cup of water to the pan. Mix well and bring it to a low simmer.

2. Add the salmon fillets, cover with a lid and cook for about 10 minutes, until the salmon changes color.

3. While the salmon is cooking, mix the vinegar, remaining olive oil, salt and ground black pepper in a large bowl. Add the spinach leaves. Mix well.

4. To serve, place some spinach leaves on each plate and top with the poached salmon.

WHITE MEAT

PARMESAN OREGANO CHICKEN SALAD

Preparation time: 10 minutes
Cooking time: 0 minutes

Serves: 2

½ pound chicken breast (grilled, diced)

2 large green bell peppers (diced)

2 tablespoons Greek yogurt

2 teaspoons fresh oregano

3 ounces Parmesan cheese (grated)

Salt to taste

Pepper to taste

NUTRITIONAL INFO (PER SERVING)
- - - - - - - - - - - - - - - - - - - -

Total Carbohydrates: 14g

Dietary Fiber: 4g

Net Carbs: 10g

Protein: 55g

Total Fat: 14g

Calories: 397

DIRECTIONS:
- -

1. Add all the ingredients except the parmesan cheese to a mixing bowl and carefully mix them together.

2. Transfer to a serving bowl or divide between two serving plates. Top with grated parmesan cheese and serve immediately.

CHICKEN WITH ALMOND CRUST

Preparation time: 10 minutes   **Serves:** 2
Cooking time: 15 minutes

Cooking oil spray
3 ounces almond flour
½ pound chicken breasts (boneless, skinless, cut into slices)
¼ cup whole milk
3 ounces mozzarella cheese (grated)
¼ teaspoon ground paprika
½ teaspoon dried parsley
Salt to taste
Pepper to taste

NUTRITIONAL INFO (PER SERVING)

Total Carbohydrates: 13g
Dietary Fiber: 6g
Net Carbs: 7g
Protein: 55g
Total Fat: 40g
Calories: 620

DIRECTIONS:

1. Preheat the oven to 400°F and grease a baking tray with cooking oil spray. Set out three plates, which will be used for preparing the chicken with three different mixtures.

2. Combine almond flour, salt and pepper. Mix well and pour on the first plate.

3. Pour whole milk on the second plate.

4. Put the grated mozzarella, paprika and dried parsley on the third plate. Mix well.

5. Dip the chicken slices into the almond flour first, then the milk, and then roll in the cheese mixture.

6. Once all of the slices are coated with all the mixtures, lay them on the greased baking tray and roast in the oven for about 15 minutes, until golden brown and totally cooked.

CHICKEN SOUP WITH CELERY

Preparation time: 10 minutes   **Serves:** 2
Cooking time: 30 minutes

1 tablespoon olive oil
1 onion (chopped)
2 celery stalks (sliced)
3 cloves garlic (minced)
5 cups all-natural chicken broth
½ pound chicken breast (boneless, skinless, cut into thin slices)
1 teaspoon garlic powder
Salt to taste
Pepper to taste

NUTRITIONAL INFO (PER SERVING)

Total Carbohydrates: 11g
Dietary Fiber: 2g
Net Carbs: 9g
Protein: 49g
Total Fat: 15g
Calories: 380

DIRECTIONS:

1. Heat the olive oil in a saucepan over a medium heat. Sauté the onion and celery for about 5 minutes or until they are soft. Add the garlic, stir and sauté for about 2 minutes, careful not to burn it.

2. Pour in the broth and bring to a boil. Reduce the heat to low, add the chicken strips, and let simmer for about 10 minutes, until the chicken is cooked through.

3. Add the garlic powder and stir to combine. Season the soup with a pinch of salt and ground black pepper. Let it simmer until everything is heated through.

4. Divide between two serving bowls. Serve immediately!

CHICKEN CUBES, INDIAN-STYLE

Preparation time: 10 minutes   **Serves:** 4
Cooking time: 15 to 20 minutes

1 bunch of fresh kale (shredded)
1 pound chicken breast (boneless, skinless, cut into cubes)
4 tablespoons olive oil
5 whole black peppercorns
4 whole cloves
3 green cardamom pods
1 onion (chopped)
2 red chilies (chopped, without seeds)
4 garlic cloves (chopped)
½ ounce fresh ginger (grated)
¼ tablespoon cumin
1 teaspoon ground coriander
1 teaspoon ground turmeric
1 ounce Greek yogurt
Salt to taste

NUTRITIONAL INFO (PER SERVING)
- - - - - - - - - - - - - - - - - - - -
Total Carbohydrates: 10g
Dietary Fiber: 2g
Net Carbs: 8g
Protein: 39g
Total Fat: 19g
Calories: 360

DIRECTIONS:

1. Add the olive oil to a large frying pan over medium heat. Sauté the peppercorns, cloves and cardamom for 2 minutes.

2. Add the chopped onion, red chilies, ginger and garlic. Sauté for a few minutes until the onions are soft.

3. Add the chicken, cumin, coriander, turmeric and salt. Stir continuously for a few minutes.

4. Once the chicken is slightly browned, add the shredded kale and season with more salt to taste.

5. Once the kale is wilted and the chicken is tender, turn off heat and add the Greek yogurt.

6. Divide between two serving plates and serve right away.

Spicy Chicken with Cheese Crust

Preparation time: 10 minutes
Cooking time: 10 minutes

Serves: 2

½ pound chicken breast (cut into steaks)
3 tablespoons olive oil
3 ounces mozzarella cheese (grated)
1 teaspoon chili powder
Salt to taste

NUTRITIONAL INFO (PER SERVING)
- -
Total Carbohydrates: 2g
Dietary Fiber: 0g
Net Carbs: 2g
Protein: 48g
Total Fat: 46g
Calories: 600

DIRECTIONS:
- -

1. Season the chicken with salt and the chili powder.

2. Add the olive oil to a frying pan and heat to medium heat.

3. Add the chicken steaks to the hot frying pan and cook for about 4 minutes on each side. Cover the steaks with cheese and flip them, quickly cook the cheese to form a crust.

4. Serve right away!

GINGER SAUTÉED CHICKEN

Preparation time: 10 minutes **Serves:** 2
Cooking time: 20 minutes

½ pound chicken breast (cut into slices)

3 teaspoons olive oil

1 tablespoon soy sauce

1 red bell pepper (thinly sliced)

1 teaspoon garlic (minced)

2 ounces fresh ginger (grated)

1 tablespoon lemon juice

2 tablespoons fresh dill (chopped)

Lemon wedges

Salt to taste

NUTRITIONAL INFO (PER SERVING)
- - - - - - - - - - - - - - - - - - - -

Total Carbohydrates: 12g

Dietary Fiber: 3g

Net Carbs: 8g

Protein: 39g

Total Fat: 12g

Calories: 305

DIRECTIONS:

1. Place the chicken in a bowl, spoon the soy sauce over and toss to coat.

2. Add 2 tablespoons of olive oil to a large frying pan over medium heat.

3. Place the chicken in the frying pan and cook for 5 minutes or until cooked through.

4. Remove from the frying pan and set aside.

5. Add the remaining oil to the same pan and keep over medium heat.

6. Add the garlic, bell pepper and ginger and cook, until lightly golden and fragrant, about 2 minutes.

7. Return the chicken to the pan and sauté for another 2 minutes.

8. Add the lemon juice. Mix well and continue cooking, stirring frequently, until the mixture is heated through.

9. Place the chicken in a serving dish, sprinkle with chopped fresh dill, season with salt and serve with lemon wedges.

SHREDDED CHICKEN WITH BROCCOLI AND CHEESE

Preparation time: 10 minutes
Cooking time: 25 minutes

Serves: 4

3 tablespoons olive oil
3 garlic cloves (minced)
½ pound broccoli (cut into pieces)
½ pound cooked chicken breast (shredded)
¼ cup chicken broth
2 ounces parmesan cheese (grated)
Small bunch parsley (finely chopped)
Salt to taste

NUTRITIONAL INFO (PER SERVING)

Total Carbohydrates: 6g
Dietary Fiber: 2g
Net Carbs: 4g
Protein: 25g
Total Fat: 16g
Calories: 260

DIRECTIONS:

1. Preheat the oven to 450°F.

2. Add the olive oil to a frying pan and place over medium-high heat.

3. Add the garlic and cook for about 2 minutes.

4. Stir in the shredded chicken and cook for about 4 minutes, until heated through. Add chicken broth, cook for about 5 minutes.

5. When it begins to boil, reduce the heat to low and cook for another 5 minutes. Remove from heat. Add the broccoli, season with salt and mix well.

6. Place the chicken mixture in a rimmed baking dish. Sprinkle grated cheese and chopped parsley over it.

7. Place in the preheated oven. Bake for about 15 minutes or until the cheese is melted.

GARLIC AND HERBS CHICKEN THIGHS

Preparation time: 10 minutes
Cooking time: 35 minutes

Serves: 4

1 pound chicken thighs
4 tablespoons olive oil
5 garlic cloves (minced)
2 tablespoons fresh oregano (chopped)
2 tablespoons fresh thyme (chopped)
Salt to taste
Pepper to taste
Fresh dill (chopped)

NUTRITIONAL INFO (PER SERVING)

Total Carbohydrates: 4g
Dietary Fiber: 2g
Net Carbs: 2g
Protein: 34g
Total Fat: 23g
Calories: 350

DIRECTIONS:

1. Preheat the oven to 350 °F.

2. Coat the chicken with the olive oil, minced garlic, fresh oregano and fresh thyme. Season with salt and pepper.

3. Place the chicken thighs on a greased baking tray. Cover with aluminum foil and transfer to the preheated oven. Roast for about 20 minutes.

4. Remove the aluminum foil and roast for about 15 minutes, until golden brown.

5. Transfer the chicken to a serving plate and garnish with fresh dill.

CHICKEN WITH ROSEMARY AND WALNUTS

Preparation time: 15 minutes
Cooking time: 20 minutes

Serves: 4

½ pound chicken breast (cut into steaks)
½ teaspoon Himalayan pink salt
Ground black pepper to taste
4 tablespoons fresh rosemary (chopped)
5 tablespoons olive oil
2 ounces walnuts (chopped)
1 onion (finely sliced)
1 teaspoon balsamic vinegar

NUTRITIONAL INFO (PER SERVING)

Total Carbohydrates: 6g
Dietary Fiber: 3g
Net Carbs: 3g
Protein: 22g
Total Fat: 29g
Calories: 350

DIRECTIONS:

1. Place the chicken breast steaks between two sheets of heavy-duty plastic wrap and pound to 1/2-inch thickness using a meat mallet or a small skillet.

2. Sprinkle the pieces with salt, black pepper and fresh rosemary.

3. Add 2 tablespoons of olive oil to a frying pan and set over medium heat.

4. Add the chicken to the hot frying pan and cook for about 5 minutes (each side) until the pieces are golden brown. Remove the chicken from the pan and place onto a plate. Cover and set aside.

5. Add the remaining oil to the frying pan and return to medium heat.

6. Add the sliced onions and cook until tender.

7. Add the cooked chicken to the frying pan, throw in the walnuts and mix.

8. Place the chicken mixture onto serving plates, drizzle with balsamic vinegar and serve!

MARINATED CHICKEN WITH CELERY

Preparation time: 15 minutes   **Serves:** 2
Cooking time: 20 minutes

½ pound chicken breast (cut into steaks)

1 teaspoon ground cumin

2 teaspoons fresh thyme (chopped)

½ cup lemon juice

½ cup celery stalks(chopped)

2 tablespoons olive oil

Ground pepper to taste

Salt to taste

NUTRITIONAL INFO (PER SERVING)

Total Carbohydrates: 3g
Dietary Fiber: 1g
Net Carbs: 2g
Protein: 38g
Total Fat: 19g
Calories: 330

DIRECTIONS:

1. Place cumin, thyme and ground pepper in a large bowl. Pour in lemon juice, stir well to combine.

2. Pour the mixture over the chicken and let it marinate in the refrigerator overnight.

3. Preheat a frying pan with olive oil over medium heat.

4. Grill the chicken steaks about 5 minutes each side, until cooked through and golden brown. Add chopped celery. Season with salt to taste.

5. Serve right away!

TOMATO AND BASIL CHICKEN SALAD

Preparation time: 5 minutes
Cooking time: 25 minutes

Serves: 4

- 5 tablespoons olive oil
- ½ pound cherry tomatoes (halved)
- 2 cups cooked chicken breast (shredded)
- 4 tablespoons basil leaves (chopped)
- 2 cups lettuce (shredded)
- 2 ounces mozzarella cheese (diced)
- Salt to taste
- Pepper to taste

NUTRITIONAL INFO (PER SERVING)

Total Carbohydrates: 4g
Dietary Fiber: 1g
Net Carbs: 3g
Protein: 29g
Total Fat: 23g
Calories: 328

DIRECTIONS:

1. Add four tablespoons of olive oil, cherry tomatoes, cooked chicken, chopped basil, lettuce and cheese to a large bowl. Season with salt and pepper. Mix well.

2. Transfer the mixture to a salad bowl. Drizzle with remaining olive oil and decorate with basil. Enjoy!

CHICKEN VEGETABLE NOODLES WITH SAGE

Preparation time: 20 minutes
Cooking time: 45 minutes

Serves: 5

2 zucchini

4 carrots

2 green bell pepper (finely sliced)

½ pound cooked chicken breast (cut into slices)

½ cup parmesan cheese (grated)

2 tablespoons sage (chopped)

4 tablespoons olive oil

Salt to taste

Pepper to taste

NUTRITIONAL INFO (PER SERVING)

Total Carbohydrates: 11g
Dietary Fiber: 4g
Net Carbs: 8g
Protein: 20g
Total Fat: 15g
Calories: 250

DIRECTIONS:

1. Wash the zucchini and carrots and run through a spiralizer to make short and thick noodles.

2. Place in a large bowl. Add the bell peppers and sage, followed by olive oil. Season with salt and pepper to taste. Mix well to combine.

3. Grease a baking dish with olive oil. Spread half of the vegetable noodles onto the baking dish, top with a layer of chicken followed by a layer of half the grated parmesan. Add the remaining vegetable noodles on top and sprinkle the remaining cheese over everything.

4. Bake 400 degrees in the oven for 40 minutes, uncovered.

5. Let it rest for about 5 minutes before serving.

GRILLED ORANGE CHICKEN

Preparation time: 10 minutes　　　　　**Serves:** 4
Cooking time: 20 minutes

1 pound chicken filets
1 tablespoon olive oil
2 teaspoons heavy cream
2 tablespoons Dijon mustard
1 tablespoon orange zest
1 tablespoon orange juice
½ teaspoon dried thyme
Black pepper to taste
Salt to taste

NUTRITIONAL INFO (PER SERVING)

Total Carbohydrates: 2g
Dietary Fiber: 0g
Net Carbs: 2g
Protein: 33g
Total Fat: 13g
Calories: 260

DIRECTIONS:

1. Place the heavy cream, mustard, thyme, orange zest, orange juice, pepper and salt in a bowl. Mix well to combine.

2. Place chicken filets in a Ziploc bag and pour the mustard mixture over them. Shake the bag to coat the chicken with the marinade.

3. Let it marinate for about 20 minutes in the fridge.

4. Heat a frying pan with olive oil. Grill the chicken over medium heat until cooked through.

Chicken with Caramelized Onion and Bell Pepper

Preparation time: 15 minutes   **Serves:** 2
Cooking time: 20 minutes

½ pound chicken breast (cut into slices)
1 red bell pepper (finely sliced)
1 onion (finely sliced)
1 teaspoon soy sauce
3 tablespoons fresh parsley (chopped)
Salt to taste
2 tablespoons rice vinegar
2 tablespoons olive oil

NUTRITIONAL INFO (PER SERVING)

Total Carbohydrates: 9g
Dietary Fiber: 3g
Net Carbs: 7g
Protein: 38g
Total Fat: 18g
Calories: 360

DIRECTIONS:
----

1. Coat a frying pan with 1 tablespoon of olive oil and set over medium heat.

2. Add the chicken slices to the hot frying pan and cook for 5 minutes, stirring, until lightly golden. Add the remaining oil to the pan and stir.

3. Add the onion, bell pepper, parsley, soy sauce and salt. Reduce the heat to low, add the vinegar and continue cooking for another 10 minutes, stirring.

4. Once the onion is caramelized (about 30 mins), remove from the heat.

5. Serve right away.

Parsley-Curry Crusted Chicken Thighs

Preparation time: 15 minutes
Cooking time: 30 minutes

Serves: 2

2 medium chicken thighs

1 egg

¼ cup almond flour

¼ teaspoon salt

½ teaspoon curry powder

Pepper to taste

4 tablespoons fresh parsley (chopped)

NUTRITIONAL INFO (PER SERVING)

Total Carbohydrates: 8g
Dietary Fiber: 4g
Net Carbs: 6g
Protein: 38g
Total Fat: 24g
Calories: 400

DIRECTIONS:

1. Preheat the oven to 425°F. Grease a baking sheet or line with parchment paper. Set aside.

2. In a mixing bowl, mix the almond flour, curry, salt, parsley and pepper.

3. In another bowl beat the egg.

4. Dip the chicken thighs into the egg, and then toss in the almond mixture to coat evenly.

5. Arrange the chicken on the prepared baking sheet and bake in the oven about 30 minutes, until cooked through.

6. Turn 2 times during the cooking to brown on both sides.

Paprika-Mustard Chicken with Spinach

Preparation time: 5 minutes
Cooking time: 20 minutes

Serves: 4

½ pound chicken breast (cut into strips)
2 cups spinach leaves
1 teaspoon smoked paprika
1 tablespoon Dijon mustard
4 tablespoons butter (divided)
2 tablespoons heavy cream
Fresh oregano (for garnish)
½ teaspoon Himalayan pink salt
Pepper to taste

NUTRITIONAL INFO (PER SERVING)

Total Carbohydrates: 3g
Dietary Fiber: 2g
Net Carbs: 2g
Protein: 38g
Total Fat: 33g
Calories: 460

DIRECTIONS:

1. Pound the chicken breast with a meat mallet until they are about ¾-inch thick.

2. Combine the paprika, salt and pepper in a shallow dish.

3. Coat the chicken evenly with the mixture.

4. Meanwhile, melt 2 tablespoons of butter in a frying pan over medium heat.

5. Cook the chicken breasts in the butter for 5 minutes per side until golden brown. Transfer the chicken to a serving plate.

6. In the same frying pan, melt remaining butter and add the spinach. Sauté for about 3 minutes.

7. In a small bowl, mix the mustard and the heavy cream.

8. To serve, place the chicken on the top of the spinach followed by the mustard.

9. Garnish with fresh oregano and enjoy.

CHICKEN WITH CAULIFLOWER, ASIAN-STYLE

Preparation time: 10 minutes
Cooking time: 20 minutes

Serves: 3

½ pound chicken breast (cut into small cubes)

2 cups cauliflower florets

2 tablespoons olive oil

1 yellow bell pepper (sliced)

1 ounce peanuts

3 garlic cloves (minced)

1½ tablespoons soy sauce

½ teaspoon hot sauce

2 tablespoons sesame seeds

Salt to taste

NUTRITIONAL INFO (PER SERVING)

Total Carbohydrates: 11g
Dietary Fiber: 4g
Net Carbs: 7g
Protein: 30g
Total Fat: 20g
Calories: 330

DIRECTIONS:

1. Place the cauliflower florets in a pot of boiling water and cook over medium heat until they are crisp-tender, about 4 minutes. Drain and set aside.

2. Heat olive oil in a large pan over medium heat. Add the chicken and cook until brown and cooked through. Transfer to a bowl and cover to keep warm.

3. Add the bell peppers to the same pan and sauté for 4 minutes. Stir in the garlic and sauté for another 2 minutes.

4. Add the cooked chicken, soy sauce, sesame seeds and hot sauce, and stir well to combine. Let the mixture simmer until it has thickened, about 3 minutes.

5. Finally, add the blanched cauliflower and peanuts and remove from the heat. Season with salt to taste.

6. Enjoy.

CHICKEN SAUTÉ WITH EGGPLANT

Preparation time: 10 minutes
Cooking time: 25 minutes

Serves: 3

½ pound chicken breast (cut into cubes)
1 medium eggplant (cut into small cubes)
1 onion (minced)
2 tablespoons olive oil
3 tablespoons butter
2 sprigs fresh sage
1 teaspoon fresh oregano (chopped)
½ teaspoon paprika
Fresh dill (chopped)
Salt to taste
Pepper to taste

NUTRITIONAL INFO (PER SERVING)

Total Carbohydrates: 13g
Dietary Fiber: 7g
Net Carbs: 7g
Protein: 27g
Total Fat: 24g
Calories: 360

DIRECTIONS:

1. Season the chicken with salt, sage, oregano, paprika and pepper.

2. Add olive oil to a frying pan and heat over medium heat.

3. Add the chicken breasts and cook for about 5 minutes, stirring, until golden brown and cooked through. Transfer to a serving plate and cover to keep warm.

4. In the same pan, melt the butter over low heat. Add the sage sprigs and cook for 1 minute. Remove the sage from the pan.

5. Add the onion and eggplant to the pan and cook in the butter for about 5 minutes, until the eggplant is cooked and the onion soft. Stir in the cooked chicken.

6. Garnish with dill and serve.

Arugula-Vinaigrette Chicken Salad

Preparation time: 10 minutes   **Serves:** 2
Cooking time: 15 minutes

Vinaigrette

  1 small onion (minced)
  ¼ teaspoon salt
  4 tablespoons olive oil
  3 tablespoons lemon juice
  ¼ cup vinegar
  Pepper to taste

Salad

  ½ pound chicken breast (cut into filets)
  2 tablespoons olive oil
  2 cups fresh arugula leaves
  ½ cups celery (diced)
  ¼ cup mozzarella cheese (diced)
  1 tomato (chopped)
  ¼ cup fresh parsley (chopped)
  Whole basil leaves (for garnish)

NUTRITIONAL INFO (PER SERVING)

Total Carbohydrates: 8g
Dietary Fiber: 2g
Net Carbs: 6g
Protein: 38g
Total Fat: 53g
Calories: 660

DIRECTIONS:

1. Pound the chicken breasts with a mallet until they are about ¼-inch thick. Heat the oil in a frying pan over medium heat. Place the chicken in the hot frying pan and brown on both sides, about 7 minutes.

2. Transfer to a plate and set side.

3. To prepare the vinaigrette, in a small bowl, mix the onion with ¼ teaspoon of salt. Whisk in 4 tablespoons of olive oil, lemon juice, vinegar and pepper until well blended.

4. To prepare the salad, place the chicken, arugula, celery, cheese, tomato and chopped parsley in a large bowl and mix well.

5. Pour the vinaigrette over, season with salt and pepper and toss well to combine.

6. Place the mixture in a salad bowl and garnish with fresh basil leaves

MEDITERRANEAN-STYLE CHICKEN SALAD

Preparation time: 10 minutes   **Serves:** 3
Cooking time: 15 minutes

½ pound chicken breast (cut into slices)
2 tablespoons balsamic vinegar
4 tablespoons extra virgin olive oil
1 tablespoon fresh oregano (chopped)
1 teaspoon fresh thyme (chopped)
3 tablespoons fresh basil (chopped)
3 cups lettuce (shredded)
1 cup cherry tomatoes (halved)
¼ cup green olives (sliced)
2 ounces goat cheese (grated)
Salt to taste
Pepper to taste

NUTRITIONAL INFO (PER SERVING)
- -
Total Carbohydrates: 7g
Dietary Fiber: 3g
Net Carbs: 5g
Protein: 29g
Total Fat: 34g
Calories: 445

DIRECTIONS:

1. Place chicken slices between 2 sheets of heavy-duty plastic wrap and pound with a mallet to about ¼-inch thick.

2. In a non-stick frying pan, heat 2 tablespoons of olive oil and brown the chicken.

3. Remove from the pan, transfer to a plate and set aside.

4. In a large bowl, mix the remaining olive oil, fresh oregano, thyme, basil, balsamic vinegar, salt and pepper.

5. In another large bowl, combine the cooked chicken, lettuce, cherry tomatoes, green olives and goat cheese.

6. Pour the dressing over the salad and toss well to combine.

7. Serve and enjoy!

CHICKEN SLICES WITH ZUCCHINI AND OLIVES

Preparation time: 10 minutes
Cooking time: 20 minutes

Serves: 2

½ pound chicken breast (cut into slices)

2 small zucchinis (cubed)

6 green olives (sliced)

2 tablespoons parmesan cheese (grated)

2 tablespoons olive oil

Salt to taste

Pepper to taste

NUTRITIONAL INFO (PER SERVING)

Total Carbohydrates: 5g
Dietary Fiber: 2g
Net Carbs: 3g
Protein: 38g
Total Fat: 26g
Calories: 405

DIRECTIONS:

1. Season chicken with salt and pepper and rub to coat.

2. Heat 1 tablespoon of olive oil in a frying pan, over medium heat and add the chicken slices.

3. Grill the chicken for about 5 minutes, until cooked through. Set aside and cover to keep warm.

4. Heat another tablespoon of olive oil in the same frying pan. Add the zucchini and olives and cook over medium heat for 5 minutes or until the zucchini is soft.

5. Serve the chicken with the zucchini mixture and sprinkle parmesan on top.

DILL CHICKEN BREAST WITH MUSHROOMS

Preparation time: 15 minutes   **Serves:** 2
Cooking time: 35 minutes

½ pound chicken breast (boneless, skinless, cut into large cubes)
¼ cup vegetable broth (divided)
3 tablespoons butter (divided)
3 tablespoons fresh dill (chopped)
½ pound fresh mushrooms (sliced)
3 tablespoons olive oil (divided)
3 tablespoons heavy cream
Salt to taste
Pepper to taste

NUTRITIONAL INFO (PER SERVING)

Total Carbohydrates: 5g
Dietary Fiber: 1g
Net Carbs: 4g
Protein: 28g
Total Fat: 34g
Calories: 420

DIRECTIONS:

1. Preheat oven to 450°F.

2. Add 1 ½ tablespoons olive oil to a large ovenproof pan and place over high heat.

3. Season the chicken with salt and pepper and add to the pan. Cook for 2 minutes until just browned. Transfer the pan to the oven.

4. Bake for 20 minutes or until chicken is cooked through. Transfer the chicken to a plate and cover to keep warm.

5. Add broth to the same pan and bring to a boil over medium heat. Scrape with a plastic spatula to remove browned bits stuck to the bottom. Reduce heat to low and let it simmer for 5 minutes.

6. Add 1 tablespoon butter, heavy cream, and dill.

7. Add the remaining olive oil and 1 tablespoon butter to a large non-stick frying pan and set over medium heat.

8. Add the mushrooms to the frying pan and sauté for 3 minutes.

9. Serve chicken with the mushrooms and the dill sauce.

PESTO STUFFED CHICKEN BREASTS

Preparation time: 15 minutes
Cooking time: 60 minutes

Serves: 4

2 chicken breasts (boneless, skinless)
3 ounces parmesan cheese
¼ cup fresh basil leaves
1 ounce walnuts
6 tablespoons extra-virgin olive oil
Salt to taste
Pepper to taste

NUTRITIONAL INFO (PER SERVING)

Total Carbohydrates: 2g
Dietary Fiber: 1g
Net Carbs: 1g
Protein: 37g
Total Fat: 37g
Calories: 483

DIRECTIONS:

1. Preheat oven to 375°F.

2. Pound chicken breasts with a meat mallet to thin and tenderize the meat.

3. In a blender or food processor, mix walnuts, 5 tablespoons olive oil and basil. Season with salt and pepper to taste.

4. Place half of the filling in the center of each chicken breast.

5. Roll up the chicken breasts tightly, tie with string on both ends.

6. Drizzle the chicken with 1 tablespoon of olive oil, season with salt and pepper to taste.

7. Place on a greased baking dish and bake in the oven for 40 minutes or until the chicken acquires golden crust and it is cooked through.

Citrus Chicken with Celery and Sesame seeds

Preparation time: 10 minutes   **Serves:** 2
Cooking time: 20 minutes

½ pound chicken filets
1 small orange (juiced and zested)
½ cup celery stalk (chopped)
2 garlic cloves (minced)
2 tablespoons sesame seeds
2 tablespoons olive oil
2 tablespoons heavy cream
Salt to taste
Pepper to taste

NUTRITIONAL INFO (PER SERVING)

Total Carbohydrates: 10g
Dietary Fiber: 3g
Net Carbs: 8g
Protein: 36g
Total Fat: 32g
Calories: 470

DIRECTIONS:

1. In a large bowl, combine the orange juice, celery, orange zest, garlic, salt and pepper. Add the chicken filets and toss well with your hands until evenly coated.

2. Preheat gas grill on high and coat the grill grates with olive oil.

3. Arrange the chicken pieces on the grate and grill for about 7 minutes, flip and cook the other side for about 7 minutes.

4. Check the doneness and if cooked through remove from the grill.

5. Place the grilled chicken into a serving dish, top with heavy cream and sesame seeds. Garnish with lemon wedges. Enjoy!

CHICKEN, TOMATO AND CARROT SOUP

Preparation time: 20 minutes   **Serves:** 4
Cooking time: 45 minutes

1 pound chicken thighs (boneless, skinless)
2 carrots (cubed)
4 ripe tomatoes (diced)
2 garlic cloves (minced)
1 onion (minced)
Pinch of curry powder
5 tablespoons fresh parsley (chopped)
3 cups chicken broth
2 cups water
2 tablespoons extra-virgin olive oil
Salt to taste
Pepper to taste

NUTRITIONAL INFO (PER SERVING)

Total Carbohydrates: 12g
Dietary Fiber: 3g
Net Carbs: 9g
Protein: 38g
Total Fat: 17g
Calories: 355

DIRECTIONS:

1. Heat the oil over medium heat. Add the onion, tomatoes, carrots and garlic. Cook for 5 minutes, stirring occasionally until the vegetables soften and the onions become translucent.

2. Stir in the parsley and cook for another minute, stirring often.

3. Add the chicken thighs, chicken broth, ½ teaspoon of salt and water. Give a stir, and bring the soup to a boil.

4. Reduce the heat to low, cover, and continue cooking for 35 minutes. Add more water if needed.

5. Remove the chicken to a bowl and let it cool. Once cooled, shred the chicken with 2 forks and set aside.

6. Add the shredded chicken to the soup followed by the curry and cook for another 5 minutes.

7. Ladle the soup into serving bowls, season with pepper and serve warm.

CREAMY CHICKEN SALAD WITH ALMONDS AND DILL

Preparation time: 20 minutes
Cooking time: 0 minutes

Serves: 3

½ pound cooked chicken breast (shredded)
2 red bell peppers (diced)
4 tablespoons heavy cream
2 ounces sliced almonds
5 tablespoons fresh dill (chopped)
1 ounce feta cheese (crumbled)
Salt to taste
Pepper to taste

NUTRITIONAL INFO (PER SERVING)

Total Carbohydrates: 13g
Dietary Fiber: 5g
Net Carbs: 8g
Protein: 32g
Total Fat: 22g
Calories: 365

DIRECTIONS:

1. Mix the cooked chicken, bell peppers, heavy cream, fresh dill and feta cheese in a bowl. Coat all ingredients well. Season with pepper and salt.

2. Transfer to a salad bowl and top with sliced almonds.

Broccoli & Olive Stuffed Chicken

Preparation time: 15 minutes
Cooking time: 30 minutes

Serves: 3

2 chicken breasts (boneless, skinless)
2 ounces parmesan cheese (grated)
½ cup broccoli (chopped)
½ small onion (minced)
4 green olives (chopped)
½ tablespoon olive oil
1 tablespoon fresh oregano (chopped)
Salt to taste
Pepper to taste

NUTRITIONAL INFO (PER SERVING)

Total Carbohydrates: 4g
Dietary Fiber: 2g
Net Carbs: 3g
Protein: 34g
Total Fat: 10g
Calories: 230

DIRECTIONS:

1. Preheat oven to 400°F.

2. Add the olive oil to a frying pan. Sauté the broccoli and the onions until soft. Stir in olives and oregano. Season with salt and pepper.

3. Halve the chicken pieces and pound with a meat mallet.

4. Place about 1 tablespoon of cheese onto each piece of chicken.

5. Then add about 2 tablespoons of the broccoli mixture and roll the chicken breasts tightly into a cylinder. Arrange them on a baking dish seam-side down.

6. Bake for 25 minutes or until the chicken is cooked through.

7. Serve warm.

Chicken Thyme Stuffed Zucchini

Preparation time: 5 minutes
Cooking time: 30 minutes

Serves: 3

1 medium zucchini (halved, seeded)
¼ pound chicken breast (cooked and shredded)
1 ounce mozzarella cheese (grated)
3 tablespoons heavy cream
4 tablespoons fresh thyme
Fresh thyme sprigs
Salt to taste
Pepper to taste

NUTRITIONAL INFO (PER SERVING)

Total Carbohydrates: 8g
Dietary Fiber: 3g
Net Carbs: 5g
Protein: 25g
Total Fat: 14g
Calories: 240

DIRECTIONS:

1. Preheat oven to 425°F.

2. Halve the zucchini and remove the seeds.

3. Place the shredded chicken, thyme and the heavy cream in a saucepan and cook over medium heat, stirring frequently, for about 3 minutes. Season with salt and pepper.

4. Spoon the mixture into halved zucchini, sprinkle with cheese and bake in the oven for about 15 minutes or until the cheese is melted and bubbly.

5. Garnish with fresh thyme sprigs and serve.

Avocado Chicken Salad with Parsley

Preparation time: 5 minutes   **Serves:** 4
Cooking time: 5 minutes

¼ pound chicken breast (cooked and shredded)

2 cups arugula leaves

1 cup lettuce (shredded)

1 ripe avocado (diced)

1 tablespoon lemon juice

4 tablespoons fresh parsley (chopped)

3 tablespoons olive oil

Salt to taste

Pepper to taste

NUTRITIONAL INFO (PER SERVING)

Total Carbohydrates: 11g

Dietary Fiber: 8g

Net Carbs: 4g

Protein: 21g

Total Fat: 43g

Calories: 490

DIRECTIONS:
----

1. Place the chicken in a bowl. Season with salt and pepper to taste.

2. Mix the olive oil and the lemon juice using a fork, the mixture should become smooth.

3. Combine the chicken, arugula leaves and shredded lettuce. Top with diced avocado.

4. Drizzle the salad with the lemon dressing. Garnish with parsley.

MUSTARD-ORANGE CHICKEN THIGHS WITH WALNUTS

Preparation time: 10 minutes
Cooking time: 30 minutes

Serves: 2

2 medium chicken thighs

3 tablespoons butter

2 tablespoons olive oil

2 tablespoons orange zest

2 tablespoons Dijon mustard

¼ cup vegetable broth

2 tablespoons heavy cream

1 ounce walnuts (chopped)

Salt to taste

Pepper to taste

NUTRITIONAL INFO (PER SERVING)
- - - - - - - - - - - - - - - - - - - -
Total Carbohydrates: 4g

Dietary Fiber: 2g

Net Carbs: 2g

Protein: 34g

Total Fat: 53g

Calories: 620

DIRECTIONS:

1. Add the butter and oil to a pan over medium heat.

2. Season the chicken with salt and pepper, coat evenly.

3. Increase the heat to high and place the thighs in the pan. Brown for 3 minutes per side. Reduce the heat, add vegetable broth, cover and cook for 20 minutes, or until cooked through.

4. Transfer to a plate and cover to keep warm.

5. Add the mustard and the heavy cream to the same pan and heat over medium heat. Using a plastic or wooden spatula, scrape sides and bottom of pan to loosen browned bits. Turn off the heat and stir in the orange zest.

6. Serve chicken drizzled with sauce. Garnish with walnuts.

RED MEAT

HAM WITH BROCCOLI AND PARMESAN

Preparation time: 15 minutes
Cooking time: 15 minutes

Serves: 2

½ pound broccoli (chopped)
6 ounces cooked ham (diced)
4 ounces parmesan cheese (grated)
1 garlic clove (minced)
¼ bunch fresh parsley (chopped)
3 tablespoons butter
Salt to taste
Pepper to taste

NUTRITIONAL INFO (PER SERVING)

Total Carbohydrates: 14g
Dietary Fiber: 5g
Net Carbs: 10g
Protein: 36g
Total Fat: 41g
Calories: 545

DIRECTIONS:

1. Add 2 tablespoons of butter to a large frying pan and place over medium heat.

2. Once the butter is hot, add the garlic and the ham and cook for about 3 minutes, until the ham is lightly browned.

3. Add the broccoli and sauté for about 3 minutes.

4. Stir in the parmesan cheese, remaining butter and parsley. Cook until the cheese is melted. Season with salt and pepper to taste.

5. Place the broccoli mixture into a serving dish and serve right away!

SAGE PORK RIBS WITH BELL PEPPER

Preparation time: 10 minutes
Cooking time: 40 minutes

Serves: 2

½ pound pork ribs
4 tablespoons fresh sage (chopped)
3 tablespoons butter
2 bell peppers (seeded, chopped)
Salt to taste
Pepper to taste

NUTRITIONAL INFO (PER SERVING)

Total Carbohydrates: 10g
Dietary Fiber: 4g
Net Carbs: 5g
Protein: 31g
Total Fat: 38g
Calories: 199

DIRECTIONS:

1. Preheat oven to 400°F. Grease a baking pan with butter.

2. Season pork ribs with salt and pepper to taste.

3. Heat the butter in a large frying pan over medium heat. Add the pork ribs and quickly brown them.

4. Transfer the pork ribs to the greased baking pan. Sprinkle with sage and chopped bell peppers.

5. Cover the baking pan with aluminum foil. Bake for about 25 minutes. Remove the foil and bake for 5 additional minutes or until the bell peppers are browned.

6. Serve right away!

BEEF AND MUSHROOM RAGU

Preparation time: 10 minutes

Cooking time: 35 minutes

Serves: 2

½ pound ground beef

½ pound fresh white mushrooms (sliced)

4 ripe tomatoes (seeded and chopped)

2 tablespoons fresh basil (chopped)

¼ cup vegetable broth

3 tablespoons olive oil

Salt to taste

Pepper to taste

NUTRITIONAL INFO (PER SERVING)

Total Carbohydrates: 14g

Dietary Fiber: 4g

Net Carbs: 10g

Protein: 42g

Total Fat: 29g

Calories: 480

DIRECTIONS:

1. Heat olive oil in a large pan over medium heat. Add the ground beef and cook for about 8 minutes or until browned, stirring frequently.

2. Add the tomatoes and cook for about 5 minutes, stirring.

3. Add vegetable broth. Reduce the heat to low and cook for about 20 minutes. Add more liquid if needed.

4. Add in sliced mushrooms and cook until they change texture. Turn off the heat, season with salt and pepper to taste.

5. Garnish with chopped basil, serve and enjoy!

CREAMY PORK TENDERLOIN WITH CHIVES

Preparation time: 10 minutes
Cooking time: 25 minutes

Serves: 2

½ pound pork tenderloin (cut into strips)
1 onion (chopped)
1 garlic clove (minced)
¼ cup vegetable broth
½ cup heavy cream
4 tablespoons fresh chives (chopped)
1 pinch ground cumin
1 pinch ground turmeric
2 tablespoons butter
Salt to taste
Pepper to taste

NUTRITIONAL INFO (PER SERVING)

Total Carbohydrates: 7g
Dietary Fiber: 2g
Net Carbs: 6g
Protein: 31g
Total Fat: 26g
Calories: 385

DIRECTIONS:
----

1. Add butter to a large frying pan and place over medium heat.

2. Once the butter is hot, add the pork and cook for about 3 minutes, until browned.

3. Stir in garlic and onion. Sauté for about 5 minutes.

4. Stir in vegetable broth, turmeric, cumin, salt and pepper. Cook over low heat for about 15 minutes or until the broth is evaporated.

5. Finally, add heavy cream and chopped chives. Then cook for additional 2 minutes.

6. Serve right away!

Sirloin and Garlic Stir Fry with Cherry Tomatoes

Preparation time: 15 minutes
Cooking time: 20 minutes

Serves: 2

½ pound sirloin steak (cubed)
4 garlic cloves (minced)
4 tablespoons fresh oregano (chopped)
4 oz. cherry tomatoes (halved)
3 tablespoons olive oil
Salt to taste
Pepper to taste

NUTRITIONAL INFO (PER SERVING)

Total Carbohydrates: 10g
Dietary Fiber: 5g
Net Carbs: 6g
Protein: 36g
Total Fat: 29g
Calories: 437

DIRECTIONS:

1. Heat olive oil in a frying pan over medium heat. Add the sirloin and cook until brown, stirring frequently.

2. Stir in the garlic and cook until golden brown. Season with salt and pepper to taste.

3. Then transfer the mixture to serving plates.

4. Sprinkle with fresh oregano and serve with cherry tomatoes.

STUFFED MEATBALLS WITH MUSTARD SAUCE

Preparation time: 15 minutes
Cooking time: 45 minutes

Serves: 3

For the meatballs

- ½ pound ground beef
- 3 ounces mozzarella cheese (cubed)
- 1 teaspoon paprika
- ¼ teaspoon ground cumin
- 1 tablespoon olive oil
- Salt to taste
- Pepper to taste

For the mustard sauce

- ½ cup heavy cream
- 4 tablespoons Dijon mustard
- 4 tablespoons fresh parsley (chopped)
- Salt to taste
- Pepper to taste

NUTRITIONAL INFO (PER SERVING)

Total Carbohydrates: 4g
Dietary Fiber: 1g
Net Carbs: 3g
Protein: 32g
Total Fat: 23g
Calories: 350

DIRECTIONS:

1. Preheat oven to 375°F.

2. To make the meatballs, add the ground beef, paprika, cumin, salt and pepper to a bowl and mix well to combine. Shape the mixture into small balls, stuffing cheese into meatballs. Set aside.

3. Grease a baking pan with olive oil, place meatballs on it.

4. Bake in the preheated oven for about 20 minutes or until golden brown.

5. To prepare the mustard sauce, heat heavy cream over low heat for about 3 minutes. Turn off heat, then stir in Dijon mustard, parsley, salt and pepper.

6. Serve the meatballs covered with the sauce. Enjoy!

STEAK SALAD WITH ALMONDS AND OREGANO

Preparation time: 20 minutes
Cooking time: 10 minutes

Serves: 3

½ pound sirloin steak (thinly sliced)
2 cups lettuce (shredded)
1 cup arugula leaves
1 pinch paprika
2 ounces almonds (chopped)
3 tablespoons fresh oregano (chopped)
1 tablespoon soy sauce
4 tablespoons olive oil
Salt to taste
Pepper to taste

NUTRITIONAL INFO (PER SERVING)

Total Carbohydrates: 6g
Dietary Fiber: 3g
Net Carbs: 3g
Protein: 28g
Total Fat: 33g
Calories: 420

DIRECTIONS:

1. Heat 2 tablespoons of olive oil in a large frying pan and cook sirloin slices until golden brown. Season with paprika, salt and pepper. Set aside.

2. In a large bowl, mix lettuce, almonds and arugula. Set aside.

3. In a small bowl, whisk soy sauce, oregano and remaining olive oil until smooth.

4. Add the cooked sirloin slices and the soy sauce mixture to the large bowl. Toss well to combine with the leaves.

5. Serve immediately!

CURRY PORK WITH CAULIFLOWER SAUCE

Preparation time: 15 minutes
Cooking time: 20 minutes

Serves: 2

½ pound pork loin (thinly sliced)
3 cups cauliflower (florets)
½ cup heavy cream
2 garlic cloves (minced)
½ teaspoon curry powder
2 tablespoons butter
Salt to taste
Pepper to taste

NUTRITIONAL INFO (PER SERVING)

Total Carbohydrates: 10g
Dietary Fiber: 4g
Net Carbs: 6g
Protein: 35g
Total Fat: 38g
Calories: 523

DIRECTIONS:

1. Season pork loin with curry, salt and pepper.

2. Add 1 tablespoon of butter to a frying pan and melt over medium heat. Place pork in frying pan and sauté for about 5 minutes. Remove from frying pan and set aside.

3. Heat remaining butter in the same frying pan and sauté garlic until slightly brown.

4. Add in the cauliflower, sauté until tender, add a little water if needed.

5. Stir in the heavy cream, salt and pepper. Cook over medium heat for about 5 minutes. Transfer this mixture to a food processor and blend until creamy.

6. Place the pork loin slices in serving plates and top with the cauliflower sauce.

7. Serve warm!

BEEF RIBS IN SPICY SAUCE

Preparation time: 20 minutes   **Serves:** 2
Cooking time: 50 minutes

½ pound beef ribs
1 onion (sliced)
4 ripe tomatoes (chopped)
2 red bell peppers (seeded, chopped)
1 cup vegetable broth
¼ bunch fresh parsley (chopped)
1 teaspoon paprika
¼ teaspoon chili powder
2 tablespoons olive oil
Salt to taste
Pepper to taste

NUTRITIONAL INFO (PER SERVING)

Total Carbohydrates: 12g
Dietary Fiber: 4g
Net Carbs: 8g
Protein: 37g
Total Fat: 15g
Calories: 335

DIRECTIONS:

1. Season beef ribs with salt and pepper to taste.

2. Heat olive oil in a pan, add beef ribs and cook until golden brown. Then stir in onions and sauté until soft.

3. Add in tomatoes, bell peppers, paprika and chili. Sauté for about 3 minutes. Then pour in vegetable broth. Cover and cook over low heat for about 40 minutes, add more broth if needed.

4. Taste the sauce and add more salt or spices to taste.

5. Garnish with fresh parsley. Serve warm!

ROSEMARY PORK LOIN WITH SOUR CREAM AND WALNUTS

Preparation time: 15 minutes (plus time in fridge)

Cooking time: 40 minutes
Serves: 4

1 pound pork loin

5 tablespoons fresh rosemary (chopped)

8 tablespoons sour cream

2 ounces walnuts (chopped)

¼ cup olive oil

Salt to taste

Pepper to taste

NUTRITIONAL INFO (PER SERVING)

Total Carbohydrates: 5g

Dietary Fiber: 3g

Net Carbs: 3g

Protein: 35g

Total Fat: 42g

Calories: 535

DIRECTIONS:

1. Preheat oven to 375°F.

2. Mix olive oil, rosemary, salt and pepper in a bowl. Evenly coat the pork loin with this mixture.

3. Place the pork on a baking pan. Cover the pan with aluminum foil. Bake for about 30 minutes. Then remove foil and bake until golden brown.

4. Remove from oven and wait about 5 minutes to slice. Place the slices on a serving plate, top them with sour cream and sprinkle with chopped walnuts.

BELL PEPPERS IN TOMATO SAUCE, ITALIAN-STYLE

Preparation time: 20 minutes
Cooking time: 35 minutes

Serves: 4

1 yellow bell pepper (seeded and sliced)
1 red bell pepper (seeded and sliced)
1 green bell pepper (seeded and sliced)
½ onion (finely chopped)
4 ripe tomatoes (seeded and chopped)
½ cup vegetable broth
4 ounces mozzarella cheese (grated)
½ teaspoon smoked paprika
1 tablespoon fresh basil (chopped)
3 tablespoons olive oil
Salt to taste
Pepper to taste

NUTRITIONAL INFO (PER SERVING)

Total Carbohydrates: 13g
Dietary Fiber: 4g
Net Carbs: 9g
Protein: 12g
Total Fat: 17g
Calories: 240

DIRECTIONS:

1. Heat olive oil in a saucepan, add onion and sauté until golden brown.

2. Add in tomatoes, bell peppers, and smoked paprika. Sauté for about 5 minutes. Then pour in vegetable broth. Cover and cook over low heat for about 15 minutes, add more broth if needed.

3. Season with salt and pepper to taste. Then transfer the sauce to a baking pan and sprinkle with grated mozzarella and chopped basil.

4. Bake in preheated oven (400°F) for about 10 minutes or until the cheese melts.

5. Serve right away!

BAKED EGGPLANT WITH BROCCOLI AND CHEESE SAUCE

Preparation time: 25 minutes   **Serves:** 4
Cooking time: 35 minutes

1 eggplant (sliced)
2 cups broccoli (florets)
2 ounces parmesan cheese (grated)
5 ounces mozzarella cheese (grated)
1 cup heavy cream
1 tablespoon fresh oregano (chopped)
¼ cup olive oil
Salt to taste
Pepper to taste

NUTRITIONAL INFO (PER SERVING)

Total Carbohydrates: 13g
Dietary Fiber: 6g
Net Carbs: 8g
Protein: 18g
Total Fat: 32g
Calories: 390

DIRECTIONS:

1. Preheat oven to 375°F.

2. Add eggplant and broccoli to a bowl. Season with salt and pepper to taste and pour in olive oil. Toss well to combine.

3. Place vegetables on a baking pan and bake in the preheated oven for about 25 minutes or until golden brown.

4. In the meantime, prepare the cheese sauce: add heavy cream, mozzarella and parmesan to a saucepan. Cook over low heat until all the cheese is melted. Turn off heat and add oregano. Season with salt and pepper to taste.

5. Remove vegetables from oven and serve them topped with cheese sauce.

Thyme-Lemon Zucchini with Feta Cheese and Almonds

Preparation time: 15 minutes
Cooking time: 20 minutes

Serves: 2

4 zucchinis (cubed)
10 ounces feta cheese (cubed)
1 tablespoon fresh lemon juice
4 tablespoons fresh thyme (chopped)
2 ounces almonds (chopped)
5 tablespoons olive oil
Salt to taste
Pepper to taste

NUTRITIONAL INFO (PER SERVING)

Total Carbohydrates: 14g
Dietary Fiber: 5g
Net Carbs: 9g
Protein: 16g
Total Fat: 40g
Calories: 460

DIRECTIONS:
----

1. Heat 2 tablespoons of olive oil in a frying pan. Add zucchini and sauté until golden brown. Season with salt and pepper to taste. Set aside.

2. In a small bowl, whisk lemon juice and remaining olive oil until smooth. Set aside.

3. Mix cooked zucchini, feta cheese, almonds and thyme in a bowl. Place on serving plates and drizzle with the lemon mixture.

4. Serve immediately.

COLORED SALAD WITH NUTS

Preparation time: 15 minutes   **Serves:** 4
Cooking time: 0

3 cups lettuce (shredded)

½ red onion (thinly sliced)

½ pound cherry tomatoes (halved)

2 cups arugula leaves

1 yellow bell pepper (seeded and sliced)

1 carrot (grated)

8 tablespoons sour cream

5 tablespoons fresh parsley (chopped)

1 ounce walnuts (chopped)

1 ounce almonds (chopped)

6 ounces mozzarella cheese (grated)

Salt to taste

Pepper to taste

NUTRITIONAL INFO (PER SERVING)

Total Carbohydrates: 13g

Dietary Fiber: 4g

Net Carbs: 9g

Protein: 18g

Total Fat: 21g

Calories: 300

DIRECTIONS:

----

1. Mix lettuce, onion, cherry tomatoes, arugula, bell pepper, carrot, parsley, walnuts, almonds and mozzarella in a bowl. Season with salt and pepper to taste.

2. Place the mixture on serving plates and top with sour cream.

3. Garnish with more chopped parsley if desired. Enjoy!

BELL PEPPER AND ALMOND CUCUMBER CANAPES

Preparation time: 20 minutes
Cooking time: 0 minutes

Serves: 4

For the cucumber base

- 2 cucumbers (sliced)
- 1 teaspoon lemon juice
- 1 pinch salt

For the topping

- 1 red bell pepper (chopped)
- 8 tablespoons sour cream
- 2 ounces almonds (chopped)
- 4 ounces Gouda cheese (grated)
- 3 tablespoons fresh dill (chopped)
- Salt to taste
- Pepper to taste

NUTRITIONAL INFO (PER SERVING)

Total Carbohydrates: 13g
Dietary Fiber: 4g
Net Carbs: 10g
Protein: 13g
Total Fat: 20g
Calories: 270

DIRECTIONS:

1. Rub cucumber slices with salt and lemon juice. Set aside.

2. Combine bell pepper, sour cream, Gouda cheese and dill in a medium bowl. Season with salt and pepper to taste. Mix well.

3. Place cucumber slices on a serving plate. Top with the sour cream mixture and sprinkle with chopped almonds.

4. Serve right away.

TOMATO AND MUSHROOM SALAD WITH SWISS CHEESE

Preparation time: 10 minutes
Cooking time: 10 minutes

Serves: 2

3 tomatoes (thinly sliced)
¼ pound fresh white mushrooms (thinly sliced)
¼ pound fresh Portobello mushrooms (thinly sliced)
4 ounces Swiss cheese (thinly sliced)
4 tablespoons fresh basil leaves
3 tablespoons butter
1 tablespoon olive oil
½ teaspoon smoked paprika
Salt to taste
Pepper to taste

NUTRITIONAL INFO (PER SERVING)

Total Carbohydrates: 13g
Dietary Fiber: 3g
Net Carbs: 10g
Protein: 20g
Total Fat: 40g
Calories: 480

DIRECTIONS:

1. Heat 2 tablespoons of butter in a large frying pan. Add all mushrooms and sauté until golden brown. Season with smoked paprika, salt and pepper. Set aside.

2. Season tomato slices with salt and pepper to taste.

3. To assemble the salad, alternate tomato slices, cheese, mushrooms and basil leaves in a serving plate, starting from the center.

4. Drizzle with olive oil and serve right away.

Zucchini Noodles with Oregano Pesto

Preparation time: 20 minutes   **Serves:** 2
Cooking time: 5 minutes

For the zucchini noodles:

- 1 large zucchini (spiralized or cut into thin strips)
- 2 tablespoons butter
- Salt to taste
- Pepper to taste

For the oregano pesto

- ¼ cup olive oil
- ¼ cup fresh oregano (only leaves)
- 1 ounce walnuts
- 4 ounces parmesan cheese (grated)
- Salt to taste
- Pepper to taste

NUTRITIONAL INFO (PER SERVING)

Total Carbohydrates: 15g
Dietary Fiber: 7g
Net Carbs: 8g
Protein: 25g
Total Fat: 59g
Calories: 640

DIRECTIONS:

1. Heat butter in a large frying pan. Add zucchini noodles and sauté for about 2 minutes. Season with salt and pepper to taste. Set aside.

2. Add olive oil, oregano leaves, walnuts and parmesan to a food processor. Blend until homogeneous. Add salt and pepper to taste.

3. Pour the oregano pesto over the zucchini noodles. Mix well. Cook for about 3 minutes or until the desired temperature is reached.

4. Serve right away.

TOMATO SOUP WITH GOUDA CHEESE

Preparation time: 15 minutes **Serves:** 4
Cooking time: 30 minutes

8 ripe tomatoes
½ onion (finely chopped)
1 garlic clove (minced)
½ pound Gouda cheese (grated)
3 tablespoons fresh oregano (chopped)
4 tablespoons olive oil
1 cup vegetable broth
5 cups water
Salt to taste
Pepper to taste

NUTRITIONAL INFO (PER SERVING)

Total Carbohydrates: 13g
Dietary Fiber: 4g
Net Carbs: 9g
Protein: 17g
Total Fat: 30g
Calories: 375

DIRECTIONS:
----

1. Bring water to a boil in a large pot. Once the water is hot, add in all tomatoes and let them rest in water for about 1 minute, the water must cover the tomatoes. Remove them and wash with cold water.

2. Peel tomatoes and remove the seeds. Set aside.

3. Heat olive oil in a large frying pan. Add onions and sauté until golden brown. Then stir in garlic and sauté for about 3 minutes.

4. Stir in tomatoes and cook over medium heat for about 5 minutes. Reduce heat, add vegetable broth and cook over low heat until tomatoes are dissolved and the soup is thick.

5. Turn off heat and add grated Gouda. Season with salt and pepper to taste.

6. Serve in soup bowls and garnish with oregano. Enjoy!

Avocado-Coconut Salad with Macadamia and Cheese

Preparation time: 15 minutes
Cooking time: 0 minutes

Serves: 2

2 large avocados
¼ cup heavy cream
6 ounces mozzarella cheese (chopped)
3 ounces macadamias (chopped)
4 ounces coconut flakes
¼ teaspoon allspice
Salt to taste
Black pepper to taste

NUTRITIONAL INFO (PER SERVING)

Total Carbohydrates: 18g
Dietary Fiber: 11g
Net Carbs: 7g
Protein: 17g
Total Fat: 55g
Calories: 605

DIRECTIONS:

1. Slice the avocados after peeling and deseeding them.

2. Mix heavy cream with salt, black pepper and allspice.

3. Place avocado slices on a serving plate. Drizzle with the heavy cream mixture.

4. Sprinkle with grated mozzarella, coconut flakes and macadamias.

5. Serve right away.

EGGPLANT, ZUCCHINI, BELL PEPPER AND MOZZARELLA SKEWERS

Preparation time: 10 minutes
Cooking time: 30 minutes

Serves: 4

1 eggplant (cubed)
1 zucchini (cubed)
1 red bell pepper (seeded, cut into large pieces)
1 green bell pepper (seeded, cut into large pieces)
½ pound mozzarella cheese (cubed)
¼ cup olive oil
4 tablespoons fresh thyme (chopped)
Salt to taste
Pepper to taste

NUTRITIONAL INFO (PER SERVING)

Total Carbohydrates: 16g
Dietary Fiber: 7g
Net Carbs: 9g
Protein: 19g
Total Fat: 24g
Calories: 335

DIRECTIONS:

1. Preheat oven to 375°F.

2. Assemble the eggplant, zucchini, bell pepper and mozzarella on bamboo skewers, alternating the different kinds of vegetables. Season with salt and pepper to taste.

3. Grease a baking pan with 1 tablespoon of olive oil and place skewers on it. Drizzle with remaining olive oil and sprinkle with thyme.

4. Bake for about 30 minutes or until golden brown. Flip the skewers once or twice during the baking time.

5. Serve immediately.

ONION LAYERS WITH PARSLEY SAUCE

Preparation time: 15 minutes   **Serves:** 3
Cooking time: 25 minutes

2 onions (peeled and halved)

8 ounces Gouda cheese (grated)

½ bunch parsley (finely chopped)

½ cup heavy cream

3 tablespoons olive oil

1 pinch cayenne pepper

Salt to taste

Black pepper to taste

NUTRITIONAL INFO (PER SERVING)
- - - - - - - - - - - - - - - - - - -
Total Carbohydrates: 10g

Dietary Fiber: 2g

Net Carbs: 8g

Protein: 21g

Total Fat: 42g

Calories: 92

DIRECTIONS:

1. Preheat oven to 400°F.

2. Separate onion layers. Set aside.

3. Grease a baking pan with 1 tablespoon of olive oil and place onion layers on it.

4. Bake onions in the preheated oven for about 15 minutes.

5. In the meantime, mix heavy cream and parsley in a bowl. Season with cayenne pepper, salt and black pepper.

6. Remove onions from oven and pour heavy cream mixture over them. Sprinkle with grated Gouda cheese and return to oven for about 10 minutes or until golden brown.

7. Serve right away.

Spinach Salad with Sun-Dried Tomatoes and Olives

Preparation time: 10 minutes (plus soaking time)

Cooking time: 10 minutes
Serves: 2

6 cups fresh spinach leaves

2 ounces green olives (chopped)

4 ounces sun-dried tomatoes

1 tablespoon soy sauce

6 ounces parmesan cheese (grated)

2 tablespoons butter

2 tablespoons olive oil

6 cups water

Salt to taste

Pepper to taste

NUTRITIONAL INFO (PER SERVING)

Total Carbohydrates: 13g
Dietary Fiber: 4g
Net Carbs: 9g
Protein: 31g
Total Fat: 47g
Calories: 570

DIRECTIONS:

1. Bring water to a boil. Turn off heat, then add in sun-dried tomatoes and let them soak for about 30 minutes.

2. Drain and chop the sun-dried tomatoes.

3. Heat butter in a large frying pan. Add sun-dried tomatoes and sauté for about 3 minutes. Set aside.

4. Add spinach leaves, olives, parmesan, olive oil, soy sauce, salt and pepper to a salad bowl. Toss well to combine.

5. Sprinkle with sun-dried tomatoes.

6. Serve right away.

BAKED BROCCOLI AND SHIITAKE OMELET

Preparation time: 10 minutes   **Serves:** 2
Cooking time: 20 minutes

1 cup broccoli (chopped)
4 ounces fresh Shiitake mushrooms (chopped)
4 eggs
2 tablespoons heavy cream
4 tablespoons fresh parsley (chopped)
½ teaspoon paprika
1 tablespoon olive oil
Salt to taste
Pepper to taste

NUTRITIONAL INFO (PER SERVING)

Total Carbohydrates: 12g
Dietary Fiber: 3g
Net Carbs: 9g
Protein: 17g
Total Fat: 24g
Calories: 330

DIRECTIONS:

1. Preheat oven to 375°F.

2. Add eggs, parsley, paprika, heavy cream, salt and pepper to a bowl, mix well. Then add in broccoli and mushrooms.

3. Grease a muffin pan with olive oil. Pour the egg mixture into it.

4. Bake for about 20 minutes or until browned.

5. Serve immediately.

LEMON CUCUMBER SALAD WITH SPICY GOAT CHEESE CRISPS

Preparation time: 15 minutes
Cooking time: 20 minutes

Serves: 2

1 cucumber (thinly sliced)
6 ounces goat cheese (thinly sliced)
2 tablespoons lemon juice
4 tablespoons olive oil
1 teaspoon lemon zest
1 teaspoon fresh dill (finely chopped)
1 teaspoon sesame seeds
¼ teaspoon chili powder
Salt to taste
Pepper to taste

NUTRITIONAL INFO (PER SERVING)

Total Carbohydrates: 9g
Dietary Fiber: 1g
Net Carbs: 8g
Protein: 28g
Total Fat: 60g
Calories: 660

DIRECTIONS:

1. Preheat oven to 400°F.

2. Line a baking pan with parchment paper and place goat cheese on it. Sprinkle with chili powder.

3. Bake goat cheese until golden brown. Remove from oven and set aside to cool down.

4. Mix cucumber, lemon juice, lemon zest, dill, sesame seeds, olive oil, salt and pepper in a salad bowl.

5. Break the goat cheese crisps into medium pieces and sprinkle over the salad.

6. Serve right away to ensure crispness!

GARLIC AND CHEESE STUFFED PORTOBELLO

Preparation time: 20 minutes

Cooking time: 20 minutes

Serves: 2

6 fresh Portobello mushrooms

8 ounces mozzarella cheese (grated)

2 garlic cloves (chopped)

2 tablespoons fresh oregano (chopped)

6 tablespoons heavy cream

2 tablespoons butter

1 tablespoon olive oil

Salt to taste

Pepper to taste

NUTRITIONAL INFO (PER SERVING)

Total Carbohydrates: 8g

Dietary Fiber: 2g

Net Carbs: 6g

Protein: 24g

Total Fat: 38g

Calories: 450

DIRECTIONS:

1. Preheat oven to 375°F

2. Remove stems from mushrooms and finely chop these stems.

3. Heat butter in a frying pan, add garlic and mushroom stems. Sauté for about 3 minutes and set aside.

4. Add oregano, heavy cream, half of the mozzarella and the mushroom mixture to a bowl. Season with salt and pepper to taste.

5. Grease a baking pan with olive oil and place the mushrooms on it. Stuff the garlic mixture into them.

6. Top mushrooms with the remaining cheese.

7. Bake in the preheated oven for about 20 minutes or until golden brown.

8. Serve warm!

CREAMY CAULIFLOWER-BACON BAKE

Preparation time: 20 minutes
Cooking time: 25 minutes

Serves: 4

3 cups cauliflower florets
1/2 cup low-fat sour cream
3 tablespoons milk
2 garlic cloves (minced)
1 red onion (chopped)
1/2 cup shredded Emmentaler cheese
1 ½ ounces smoked bacon, cooked and chopped

NUTRITIONAL INFO (PER SERVING)
- -
Total Carbohydrates: 9g
Dietary Fiber: 3g
Net Carbs: 7g
Protein: 9g
Total Fat: 11g
Calories: 169

DIRECTIONS:

1. Preheat oven to 425°F.

2. Bring a pot of water to a boil.

3. Cook the cauliflower for about 4 minutes, until crisp-tender. Remove from the pot and rinse under running water. Strain the liquid (reserve ½ cup) and transfer to a bowl.

4. Mix the sour cream, milk, garlic and red onion.

5. Add the cream mixture to the veggie bowl and toss to coat. If you need some more liquid, add some of the cooking water.

6. Transfer the mixture into an ovenproof dish and spread evenly. Top with the smoked bacon and cheese.

7. Cover and bake for 25 minutes. Check if the cauliflower is tender. Remove the cover and cook for 5 minutes more to get a crispy top.

8. Take the dish out of the oven and let cool a little bit before serving.

BAKED MOZZARELLA-EGGPLANT ROUNDS

Preparation time: 5 minutes
Cooking time: 15 to 20 minutes
Serves: 4

2 medium sized eggplants
1/2 cup freshly grated Mozzarella cheese
2 garlic cloves
1 teaspoon dried oregano
Salt & freshly ground black pepper, to taste

NUTRITIONAL INFO (PER SERVING)

Total Carbohydrates: 18g
Dietary Fiber: 10g
Net Carbs: 7g
Protein: 7g
Total Fat: 3g
Calories: 112

DIRECTIONS:

1. Preheat oven to 425°F.

2. Line a baking dish with parchment paper.

3. Rinse the eggplants and pat dry. Slice into 1/4-inch thick rounds and place them on the dish.

4. Crush the garlic and spread over the eggplants. Sprinkle with oregano, salt and pepper.

5. Top the eggplant slices with grated Mozzarella and cook for 19–20 minutes, until they are soft and the cheese melts.

6. Remove from the oven and enjoy.

Zucchini Noodle Stir-Fry with Almond Chicken

Preparation time: 15 minutes

Cooking time: 30 minutes

Serves: 6

4 medium zucchinis

1 cup of chicken breast (cut into bite-sized pieces)

1 carrot (diced)

1 medium head kale (chopped)

2 chives (thinly sliced)

1 red hot chili pepper (thinly sliced)

¼ cup almonds (chopped)

¼ cup fresh parsley (chopped)

½ tablespoon grated fresh ginger root

3 tablespoon of Tamari

1 tablespoon of coconut oil for cooking (deodorized)

½ tsp of curry powder

Salt and freshly ground black pepper, to taste

NUTRITIONAL INFO (PER SERVING)

Total Carbohydrates: 9g

Dietary Fiber: 3g

Net Carbs: 7g

Protein: 12g

Total Fat: 5g

Calories: 127

DIRECTIONS:

1. Create zucchini noodles with a spiralizer.

2. Heat the coconut oil in a skillet.

3. Brown the chicken pieces on all sides.

4. Reduce the heat to medium. Add the zucchini, chili pepper, carrot, kale, chives, cilantro, ginger, and curry powder. Season with salt and pepper to taste and cook for 5–10 minutes, or until the zucchini becomes tender and the kale wilts.

5. Add the soy sauce and stir in the almonds. Cook for another 5 minutes.

6. Remove the saucepan from heat. Let rest for 10 minutes before serving.

Cucumber Salad with Toasted Sunflower Seeds

Preparation time: 15 minutes
Cooking time: 5 minutes

Serves: 4

4 cucumbers (sliced)
2 green onions (thinly sliced)
2 limes
2 scallions (finely chopped)
2 tablespoons sunflower seeds (toasted)
2 tablespoons apple cider vinegar
2 tablespoons sunflower oil
2 tablespoons parsley (chopped)
Salt and pepper, to taste

NUTRITIONAL INFO (PER SERVING)

Total Carbohydrates: 13g
Dietary Fiber: 2g
Net Carbs: 10g
Protein: 3g
Total Fat: 8g
Calories: 123

DIRECTIONS:

1. Halve the limes. Slice one half and juice the rest.

2. Cut the cucumber into slices and place in a salad bowl.

3. Add the scallions, onions, sunflower seeds and parsley. Drizzle with apple cider vinegar, olive oil and lime juice. Stir well for the flavors to combine.

4. Serve garnished with lime slices.

Quick and Easy Sea Bass Soup

Preparation time: 5 minutes
Cooking time: 15 minutes

Serves: 6

4 large zucchini
1 pound sea bass fillets, cut into strips
1 red onion (thinly sliced)
Zest and juice from one lemon
6 tablespoons coriander leaves (chopped)
1 ½ cups soy milk
1 tablespoon extra-virgin olive oil
10 ounces tomato paste
2 teaspoons curry powder

NUTRITIONAL INFO (PER SERVING)

Total Carbohydrates: 23g
Dietary Fiber: 3g
Net Carbs: 20g
Protein: 25g
Total Fat: 6g
Calories: 232

DIRECTIONS:

1. Spiralize the zucchini and set aside.

2. Heat the olive oil in a large stockpot. Sauté the onion for 4–5 minutes until translucent.

3. Add the zucchini noodles and cook for 4–6 minutes until the edges become brown.

4. Pour the soy milk then add the sea bass, lemon juice, and half of the coriander.

5. Add the tomato paste and curry powder.

6. Bring the soup to a boil, lower the heat and simmer for 10 minutes.

7. Garnish with coriander and lemon zest.

Sardine Salad with Zucchini Black Sesame Noodles

Preparation time: 15 minutes   **Serves:** 6
Cooking time: 0 minutes

4 zucchinis
10 ounces canned sardines (drained)
2 small red onions (chopped)
2 celery stalks (chopped)
¼ cup parsley (chopped)
1 tablespoon dried oregano
3 tablespoons black sesame seeds
4 tablespoons apple cider vinegar
2 tablespoons Tamari
1 inch fresh ginger root (minced or grated)
2 tablespoons extra virgin olive oil
1 teaspoon chili powder or hot pepper sauce
salt and black pepper, to taste

NUTRITIONAL INFO (PER SERVING)

Total Carbohydrates: 9g
Dietary Fiber: 3g
Net Carbs: 6g
Protein: 15g
Total Fat: 13g
Calories: 206

DIRECTIONS:

1. Spiralize the zucchinis to create the noodles.

2. Prepare the dressing by combining the soy sauce, oregano, apple cider vinegar and chili powder in a mixing bowl. Whisk in the olive oil little by little until you get a thick sauce.

3. In a large serving bowl, combine the zucchini noodles, sardines, onions, ginger, chopped celery and parsley. Coat with the dressing and top with sesame seeds to serve.

SPICY CHICKEN VEGETABLE SOUP

Preparation time: 15 minutes   **Serves:** 6
Cooking time: 30 minutes

2 carrots (sliced)

¼ cup bamboo shoots

1 red Poblano pepper (finely chopped)

2 celery stalks (chopped)

¾ pound of boneless, skinless chicken breasts (cut into bite-sized pieces)

5 cups vegetable stock

Zest and juice from 1 lime

1 cup Champignon mushrooms (chopped)

2 green onions (sliced)

1 teaspoon curry powder (or 3 curry leaves)

1 tablespoon white wine vinegar

2 tablespoons ginger powder

2 tablespoons Tamari

1 teaspoon turmeric powder

2 tablespoons dry white wine

2 tablespoons olive oil

Salt and pepper, to taste

NUTRITIONAL INFO (PER SERVING)

Total Carbohydrates: 8g
Dietary Fiber: 3g
Net Carbs: 5g
Protein: 19g
Total Fat: 9g
Calories: 195

DIRECTIONS:

1. Heat the olive oil in a large skillet over medium heat.

2. Add the spices, salt and pepper, and cook for about 1 minute.

3. Add the meat to the pan and cook for 5 minutes per side, until golden.

4. Stir in the onions, mushrooms, carrots, celery and bamboo shoots. Cook for 5 more minutes.

5. Finally, add the soy sauce, lime juice and zest, white wine vinegar, dry white wine and vegetable stock. Cover and simmer for about 25 minutes, until the veggies are soft. Serve hot.

SPICY BEEF SOUP WITH ZUCCHINI NOODLES

Preparation time: 15 minutes
Cooking time: 35 minutes

Serves: 8

3 large zucchinis (spiralized or peeled into strips)
1 pound grass-fed ground beef
2 carrots (sliced)
4 cups chicken broth
2 heads kale (chopped)
4 green onions (thinly sliced)
1 tablespoon fresh ginger (grated)
2 teaspoons chili paste
1 tablespoon sesame oil

NUTRITIONAL INFO (PER SERVING)

Total Carbohydrates: 11g
Dietary Fiber: 3g
Net Carbs: 8g
Protein: 23g
Total Fat: 6g
Calories: 191

DIRECTIONS

1. Heat a large saucepan over medium heat.

2. Brown the beef for 5–6 minutes. Remove from heat and set aside.

3. Heat the oil in the same saucepan, over medium-high heat, and add the veggies, chicken broth, kale, chili paste, ginger and onions.

4. Bring to a boil, reduce heat to low and simmer for 20 minutes, until the vegetables are soft.

5. Stir in the ground beef and continue cooking together for another 10 minutes. Serve hot.

Low Carb Chili

Preparation time: 15 minutes   **Serves:** 6
Cooking time: 60 minutes

1 ¼ pound grass-fed ground beef

3 Roma tomatoes (chopped)

2 green onions (chopped)

8 ounces canned tomatoes (chopped with juice)

1 medium green bell pepper (chopped)

1 carrot (sliced)

2 celery stalks (chopped)

1½ teaspoons ground cumin seeds

2 chili peppers (chopped)

Salt and pepper to taste

¾ cup vegetable stock, or as needed

NUTRITIONAL INFO (PER SERVING)

Total Carbohydrates: 7g

Dietary Fiber: 2g

Net Carbs: 5g

Protein: 30g

Total Fat: 6g

Calories: 209

DIRECTIONS:

1. Brown the ground beef in a large skillet for 5–6 minutes.

2. Remove the fat and season with salt and pepper.

3. Add the onions and bell pepper to the ground beef and cook for 2 minutes more.

4. Stir in the Roma tomatoes, carrot, celery, and canned tomatoes. Mix well. Add the water and bring to a boil.

5. Reduce the heat to low, add the cumin seeds and chili peppers and allow to simmer for about 90–120 minutes, until slightly thickened, stirring occasionally.

6. Serve hot.

BREAKFAST RECIPES

PIZZA WITH OLIVES, MUSHROOMS, AND BACON

Preparation time: 10 minutes
Cooking time: 20 to 25 minutes

Serves: 2

2 medium eggs (well beaten)
10 cherry tomatoes (halved)
1 large Champignon mushroom (sliced)
6 slices of bacon (cooked)
8 Kalamata olives (thinly sliced)
½ teaspoon dried oregano
1 ounce low-fat Mozzarella (cubed)
2 teaspoons olive oil
Basil leaves to garnish
Salt and freshly ground pepper, to taste

NUTRITIONAL INFO (PER SERVING)

Total Carbohydrates: 17g
Dietary Fiber: 5g
Net Carbs: 12g
Protein: 17g
Total Fat: 18g
Calories: 285

DIRECTIONS:

1. Preheat oven to 350°F.

2. Beat the eggs, season with salt, pepper, and oregano, and set aside.

3. Heat some olive oil in a medium heatproof skillet. Once hot, add the eggs and cook for 2 minutes until the mixture comes together.

4. Evenly spread half of the tomatoes, olives, mushrooms and bacon on top of the eggs. Top with a third of the cheese. Repeat for the next layer and add the remaining cheese on top. Cook for about 3 minutes until cheese begins to melt.

5. Transfer to the oven and bake for 3–4 minutes until the cheese becomes golden brown.

6. Remove from the oven and serve while hot.

CHEESY NO-BAKED FRITTATA

Preparation time: 10 minutes   **Serves:** 6
Cooking time: 20 minutes

6 eggs
1 tablespoon coconut oil for cooking (deodorized)
1 garlic clove (minced)
1 medium yellow bell pepper (chopped)
2 green onions (chopped)
2 (14-ounce) cans diced tomatoes
3 ½ ounces Parmesan cheese
2 tablespoons tomato paste
1 chili (chopped)
1 teaspoon cumin
1 teaspoon turmeric
Pinch of cayenne pepper
Salt and pepper to taste
Small bunch of fresh coriander to serve

NUTRITIONAL INFO (PER SERVING)

Total Carbohydrates: 10g
Dietary Fiber: 3g
Net Carbs: 7g
Protein: 13g
Total Fat: 11g
Calories: 179

DIRECTIONS:

1. Heat the coconut oil in a large skillet. Add the chopped onion and garlic and sauté for 3–4 minutes until fragrant and soft.

2. Add the bell peppers and cook for 5 minutes more, until tender.

3. Stir in the tomatoes and tomato paste and stir well. Add the chili and the spices (cumin, turmeric and cayenne pepper) and simmer for 5 minutes. Adjust the taste if necessary. Bring the cheese to the pan. Stir to mix well.

4. Crack the eggs over the tomato mixture, making sure they are evenly distributed. Simmer for 10–15 minutes more, covered. Check from time to time to see if the mixture doesn't get burn. If you want the eggs well done, cook for 15 minutes.

5. Garnish with fresh coriander and serve.

KALE AND EGGS BENEDICT

Preparation time: 15 minutes
Cooking time: 10 minutes

Serves: 1

2 large eggs
1 tablespoon cream cheese
1 garlic clove (peeled and crushed)
½ butter
2 teaspoons coconut oil
3 ounces baby spinach
Salt and pepper to taste

NUTRITIONAL INFO (PER SERVING)

Total Carbohydrates: 5g
Dietary Fiber: 2g
Net Carbs: 3g
Protein: 16g
Total Fat: 23g
Calories: 280

DIRECTIONS:

Kale and egg

1. Melt 1 teaspoon coconut oil in a large skillet. Sauté the garlic for 2–3 minutes until golden brown.

2. Add the spinach.

3. Cook for 5 minutes, covered. Remove from heat but leave the cover on.

4. Melt 1 more teaspoon of coconut oil in another skillet.

5. Crack 1 egg and separate the white from the yolk. Crack the other whole egg in the bowl with the egg white. Add these eggs to the skillet and cook for 2 minutes.

Hollandaise Sauce

6. Meanwhile, melt the cream cheese to form a creamy sauce.

7. Blend the remaining egg yolk in a food processor for 20 seconds and add some salt and pepper. Then begin to add the butter and cream cheese mixture about a quarter at a time while continuously blending until smooth.

8. Serve the eggs on a bed of spinach leaves, topped with sauce.

KALE, ZUCCHINI AND GOAT CHEESE CRUSTLESS QUICHE

Preparation time: 15 minutes
Cooking time: 45 minutes

Serves: 4

4 large eggs
8 ounces fresh zucchinis, sliced
10 ounces kale
3 garlic cloves (minced)
1 cup soy milk
1 ½ ounces goat cheese
¼ cup grated parmesan
½ cup shredded cheddar cheese
2 teaspoons olive oil
Salt & pepper, to taste

NUTRITIONAL INFO (PER SERVING)

Total Carbohydrates: 15g
Dietary Fiber: 2g
Net Carbs: 13g
Protein: 19g
Total Fat: 18g
Calories: 290

DIRECTIONS:

1. Preheat oven to 350°F.

2. Heat 1 teaspoon olive oil in a skillet over medium-high heat. Sauté the garlic for 1 minute until fragrant.

3. Add the zucchinis and cook for 5–7 minutes more until soft.

4. Beat the eggs, and then add the milk and Parmesan cheese little by little.

5. Meanwhile heat the remaining olive oil in another skillet and add the kale. Cover and cook for about 5 minutes until it wilts.

6. Slightly grease a baking dish with cooking spray and spread the kale leaves across the bottom. Add the zucchinis and top with goat cheese.

7. Pour the egg, milk and parmesan mixture evenly over the other ingredients. Top with cheddar cheese.

8. Bake for 50–60 minutes until golden brown. Check the center of the quiche, it should have a solid consistency.

9. Let chill for a few minutes before serving.

SPAGHETTI SQUASH CARBONARA

Preparation time: 15 minutes

Cooking time: 20 minutes

Serves: 4

1 small spaghetti squash

6 ounces bacon (roughly chopped)

1 large tomato (sliced)

2 chives (chopped)

1 garlic clove (minced)

6 ounces low-fat cottage cheese

1 cup Gouda cheese (grated)

2 tablespoons olive oil

Salt and pepper, to taste

NUTRITIONAL INFO (PER SERVING)

Total Carbohydrates: 11g

Dietary Fiber: 0g

Net Carbs: 11g

Protein: 18g

Total Fat: 21g

Calories: 305

DIRECTIONS:

1. Preheat the oven to 350°F.

2. Cut the spaghetti squash in half, brush with some olive oil and bake for 20–30 minutes, skin side up. Remove from the oven and remove the core with a fork, creating the spaghetti.

3. Heat one tablespoon of olive oil in a skillet. Cook the bacon for about 1 minute until crispy.

4. Quickly wipe out the pan with paper towels.

5. Heat another tablespoon of oil and sauté the garlic, tomato and chives for 2–3 minutes. Add the spaghetti and sauté for another 5 minutes, stirring occasionally to keep from burning.

6. Begin to add the cottage cheese, about 2 tablespoons at a time. If the sauce becomes too thick, add about ¼ cup water. The sauce should be creamy, but not too runny or thick. Allow to cook for another 3 minutes.

7. Serve immediately.

HIGH-PROTEIN GLUTEN-FREE PANCAKES

Preparation time: 5 minutes
Cooking time: 10 minutes

Serves: 2

6 eggs
1 cup low-fat cream cheese
1 ½ teaspoons baking powder
1 scoop protein powder
¼ cup almond meal
½ teaspoon salt

NUTRITIONAL INFO (PER SERVING)

Total Carbohydrates: 9g
Dietary Fiber: 1g
Net Carbs: 8g
Protein: 31g
Total Fat: 14g
Calories: 288

DIRECTIONS

1. Combine the dry ingredients in a food processor. Add the eggs one by one, and then the cream cheese. Process until you get a batter.

2. Slightly grease a skillet with cooking spray and place over medium-high heat.

3. Ladle the batter into the skillet. Gently rotate the skillet to create round pancakes.

4. Cook for about 2 minutes on each side.

5. Serve pancakes with your favorite topping.

HIGH-PROTEIN BREAKFAST

Preparation time: 2 minutes
Cooking time: 3 minutes

Serves: 2

3 tablespoons chia seeds

3 tablespoons flax seeds

2 ounces coconut flour

1 cup soy milk

⅔ cup water

½ tablespoon ground cinnamon

Pinch of nutmeg

2 scoops of vanilla protein powder

NUTRITIONAL INFO (PER SERVING)

Total Carbohydrates: 23g

Dietary Fiber: 10g

Net Carbs: 13g

Protein: 31g

Total Fat: 20g

Calories: 405

DIRECTIONS:

1. Combine all the ingredients and set aside for the night. It is best to keep the bowl in the fridge.

2. In the morning, bring the soaked ingredients to a simmer and cook until the mixture thickens. You can also enjoy it without cooking, to fully benefit from all the vitamins and minerals in the ingredients.

3. Serve with your favorite topping.

FLAXSEED CREPES WITH YOGURT

Preparation time: 3 minutes
Cooking time: 2 minutes
Serves: 2

8 large egg whites
½ cup plain yogurt
4 tablespoons ground flaxseeds
½ cup soy milk

DIRECTIONS:

1. Combine the flaxseeds with the milk and mix well until smooth and free of lumps.

2. Beat the egg white and add to the flaxseeds mixture little by little.

3. Slightly grease a non-stick skillet with cooking spray. Ladle the batter and cook for about 60–90 seconds on one side and 10–15 seconds on the other.

4. Top with yogurt and serve.

HERB CHICKEN BURGER

Preparation time: 5 minutes   **Serves:** 4
Cooking time: 20 minutes

4 large eggs
1 ½ pounds ground chicken thighs (skinless, boneless)
4 slices bacon (chopped)
1 green onion (chopped)
Small bunch of dill (chopped)
8 slices gluten-free toast
2 ½ teaspoons olive oil
1 large tomato (sliced)
Salt and pepper to taste

NUTRITIONAL INFO (PER SERVING)

Total Carbohydrates: 22g
Dietary Fiber: 4g
Net Carbs: 18g
Protein: 63g
Total Fat: 35g
Calories: 599

DIRECTIONS:

1. In a bowl, combine the chopped bacon and ground chicken. Add the onion and dill and stir well. Season with black pepper and salt. Shape the mixture into patties about ¾ inch thick. Wrap in plastic and leave in the fridge for half an hour to harden.

2. Heat the grill to a medium-high heat and grease with cooking spray. Place the chicken burgers on the grill. Grill for 8 minutes each side (until not pink inside).

3. Place the toast slices in the toaster and heat a little bit.

4. Heat the olive oil in a skillet over medium-high heat and fry the eggs for at least 3 minutes.

5. Assemble the burger: place a toast slice, the chicken patty, a tomato slice, the egg, and another toast slice.

COTTAGE CHEESE OMELET WITH VEGGIES

Preparation time: 3 minutes
Cooking time: 5 minutes

Serves: 2

5 eggs (beaten)
1 red onion (chopped)
1 cup kale (chopped)
¾ cup ricotta cheese
1 large tomato (sliced)
Cooking oil spray

NUTRITIONAL INFO (PER SERVING)

Total Carbohydrates: 18g
Dietary Fiber: 3g
Net Carbs: 15g
Protein: 27g
Total Fat: 19
Calories: 343

DIRECTIONS:

1. Heat a non-stick skillet over medium-high heat.

2. Add the eggs, tilting the skillet to ensure an even layer. Next, add the red onion over the omelet.

3. Cook for 1–2 minutes, and add 1/2 of the ricotta cheese, kale, and tomato slices on half of the omelet. Cook for about 2 minutes more. Flip the naked half of the omelet onto the other half to make a perfect half circle.

4. Serve with the remaining ricotta cheese.

DESSERTS

Coconut and almond Squares

Preparation time: 10 minutes
Cooking time: 25 minutes

Serves: 12

1 cup coconut flour

½ cup melted butter

2 cups almonds

½ cup shredded coconut

¼ cup agave syrup

½ cup ground chia seeds

¼ teaspoon liquid stevia

NUTRITIONAL INFO (PER SERVING)

Total Carbohydrates: 19g
Dietary Fiber: 14g
Net Carbs: 6g
Protein: 8g
Total Fat: 28g
Calories: 353

DIRECTIONS:

1. Preheat the oven to 350°F. Bake the almonds on a baking dish for 6–8 minutes. Set aside to cool.

2. Place the almonds on one half of a piece of parchment paper and fold the other half over. Crush the almonds with a rolling pin or a kitchen hammer.

3. Combine the ground chia seeds with shredded coconut and coconut flour.

4. Add the crushed almonds and stir.

5. Stir in the butter, agave syrup, and stevia and mix until you form a dough.

6. Place the dough in a baking dish lined with parchment paper.

7. Bake at for about 25 minutes and remove from the oven.

8. Let cool, and then refrigerate for 120 minutes.

9. Cut into squares and serve.

WALNUT AND PISTACHIO COOKIES

Preparation time: 10 minutes
Cooking time: 10 minutes
Serves: 20

2 cups walnuts
1 cup coconut oil
3 tablespoons erythritol
1 cup pistachios (de-shelled)
1 teaspoon vanilla extract

NUTRITIONAL INFO (PER SERVING)

Total Carbohydrates: 2g
Dietary Fiber: 1g
Net Carbs: 1g
Protein: 4g
Total Fat: 20g
Calories: 188

DIRECTIONS:

1. Grind the pecans and pistachios in a food processor until they turn into a flour.

2. Add the other ingredients to the food processor and blend until you get a dough.

3. Roll the dough into a cylinder and cover with parchment paper.

4. Refrigerate for about 3 hours.

5. Remove from the fridge and slice into ½ inch slices.

6. Preheat oven to 325°F.

7. Place the slices on a baking sheet.

8. Cook for about 10 minutes until golden brown.

COCOA PUDDING WITH CHIA SEEDS

Preparation time: 20 minutes
Cooking time: 5 minutes

Serves: 2

2 tablespoons cocoa powder

1 almond milk

⅓ cup chia seeds

⅓ cup heavy whipping cream

Seeds from 1 vanilla pod

1 tablespoon erythritol

2 tablespoons cocoa nibs

NUTRITIONAL INFO (PER SERVING)

Total Carbohydrates: 11g

Dietary Fiber: 6g

Net Carbs: 3g

Protein: 4g

Total Fat: 28g

Calories: 284

DIRECTIONS:

1. Bring the water to a boil and add the cocoa powder. Stir well to combine. Set aside to cool a little bit.

2. In a bowl, whisk together the whipping cream, cooled cocoa, vanilla seeds and erythritol.

3. Add the chia seeds and cocoa nibs.

4. Transfer to a small bowl and refrigerate for a minimum of 60 minutes before serving.

CHOCOLATE BANANA MINI TARTS

Preparation time: 15 minutes
Cooking time: 8 minutes

Serves: 4

Crust

    2 large egg whites
    2 tablespoons coconut flour
    1 tablespoons erythritol
    ¼ cup chia seeds

Filling

    4 tablespoons almond butter
    2 tablespoons coconut oil

Top

    4 tablespoons carob powder
    ¼ cup erythritol
    1 ripe bananas
    2 tablespoons half-and-half
    1 vanilla pod
    ½ teaspoon cinnamon
    Pinch of nutmeg

NUTRITIONAL INFO (PER SERVING)

Total Carbohydrates: 16g
Dietary Fiber: 4g
Net Carbs: 12g
Protein: 6g
Total Fat: 25g
Calories: 289

DIRECTIONS:

1. Preheat the oven to 350°F.

2. Grind the chia seeds in a food processor until they resemble flour.

3. Add the coconut flour, erythritol, and egg whites into the chia seed powder and process until combined.

4. Divide the mixture into 4 and cover the bottom of some small tart tins. Bake for about 8 minutes.

5. Melt together the almond butter and coconut oil.

6. After the crust is ready, let cool a little bit and cover with the coconut oil-butter mixture. Put in the fridge for 30 minutes.

7. Meanwhile, mash the banana and combine with carob powder, erythritol, the seeds from the vanilla pod, cinnamon, nutmeg and half-and-half. Blend until smooth and creamy.

8. Remove the tarts from the fridge, top with the blended banana mixture and return to the fridge for at least an hour before serving.

CREAMY CHOCOLATE BROWNIES

Preparation time: 20 minutes   **Serves:** 8
Cooking time: 20 minutes

Brownies

- ½ cup coconut flour
- 2 eggs
- ½ tsp liquid Stevia
- ⅓ cup erythritol
- ⅓ cup cocoa powder
- 3 teaspoons lemon juice
- 2 ounces butter
- 3 tablespoons ground flaxseeds
- ¼ teaspoon baking soda
- 2 ounces dark chocolate, no sugar added (broken into pieces)

Chocolate Cream

- 1 ounce dark chocolate, no sugar added (broken into small pieces)
- ¼ cup fat-free half-and-half
- 1 tablespoon coconut oil

NUTRITIONAL INFO (PER SERVING)
- - - - - - - - - - - - - - - - - - - -
Total Carbohydrates: 7g
Dietary Fiber: 3g
Net Carbs: 4g
Protein: 5g
Total Fat: 18g
Calories: 202

DIRECTIONS:

1. Preheat the oven to 350°F.
2. Grease a small baking dish with cooking spray or line with parchment paper.
3. Combine the chocolate with the butter and melt over simmering water.
4. Whisk in the egg and combine with stevia and erythritol. Slowly add to the chocolate mixture.
5. Stir in the dry ingredients one by one.
6. Transfer the batter to the baking dish and cook for 25–30 minutes. Let cool before cutting into pieces.
7. Combine all the ingredients for the cream and bring to a simmer.
8. Spread over the brownie and keep in the fridge before serving.

84825900R00095

Made in the USA
Middletown, DE
21 August 2018